T0202379

The EHRA Book of
Pacemaker, ICD, and CRT Troubleshooting

EUROPEAN SOCIETY OF CARDIOLOGY PUBLICATIONS PORTFOLIO

The ESC Textbook of Cardiovascular Medicine (Third Edition)
Edited by A. John Camm, Thomas F. Lüscher, Gerald Maurer, and Patrick W. Serruys

The ESC Textbook of Intensive and Acute Cardiovascular Care (Second Edition)
Edited by Marco Tubaro, Pascal Vranckx, Susanna Price, and Christiaan Vrints

The ESC Textbook of Cardiovascular Imaging (Second Edition)
Edited by Jose Luis Zamorano, Jeroen Bax, Juhani Knuuti, Patrizio Lancellotti, Luigi Badano, and Udo Sechtem

The ESC Textbook of Preventive Cardiology
Edited by Stephan Gielen, Guy De Backer, Massimo Piepoli, and David Wood

The EHRA Book of Pacemaker, ICD, and CRT Troubleshooting: Case-based learning with multiple choice questions (Volume 2)
Edited by Harran Burri, Carsten Israel, and Jean-Claude Deharo

The EACVI Echo Handbook
Edited by Patrizio Lancellotti and Bernard Cosyns

The ESC Handbook of Preventive Cardiology: Putting prevention into practice
Edited by Catriona Jennings, Ian Graham, and Stephan Gielen

The EACVI Textbook of Echocardiography (Second Edition)
Edited by Patrizio Lancellotti, Jose Luis Zamorano, Gilbert Habib, and Luigi Badano

The EHRA Book of Interventional Electrophysiology: Case-based learning with multiple choice questions
Edited by Hein Heidbuchel, Matthias Duytschaever, and Harran Burri

The ESC Textbook of Vascular Biology
Edited by Robert Krams and Magnus Back

The ESC Textbook of Cardiovascular Development
Edited by Jose Maria Perez Pomares and Robert Kelly

The ESC Textbook of Cardiovascular Magnetic Resonance
Edited by Sven Plein, Massimo Lombardi, Steffen Petersen, Emanuela Valsangiacomo, Chiara Bucciarelli-Ducci, and Victor Ferrari

The ESC Textbook of Sports Cardiology
Edited by Antonio Pelliccia, Heid Heidbuchel, Domenico Corrado, Mats Borjesson, and Sanjay Sharma

The ESC Handbook of Cardiac Rehabilitation
Edited by Ana Abreu, Massimo Piepoli, and Jean-Paul Schmid

The ESC Textbook of Intensive and Acute Cardiovascular Care (Third Edition)
Edited by Marco Tubaro, Pascal Vranckx, Susanna Price, Christiaan Vrints, and Eric Bonnefoy

The ESC Textbook of Cardiovascular Imaging (Third Edition)
Edited by Jose Luis Zamorano, Jeroen Bax, Juhani Knuuti, Patrizio Lancellotti, Bogdan Popescu, and Fausto Pinto

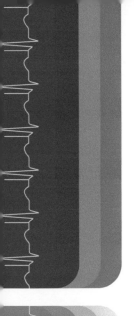

The EHRA Book of
Pacemaker, ICD, and CRT Troubleshooting

Case-based learning with multiple choice questions

Volume 2

Prof. Haran Burri FEHRA

EHRA treasurer, former EHRA Education Committee chairman
Director, Cardiac Pacing Unit
Cardiology Department
University Hospital of Geneva, Switzerland

Assoc. Prof. Jens Brock Johansen PHD

Former co-chair (CP) EHRA Certification Committee
Director, Cardiac Pacing Unit
Cardiology Department
Odense University Hospital, Denmark

Prof. Nicholas J. Linker BSC, MD, FRCP, ECDS, FACC, FESC, FHRS

Former co-chair (CP) EHRA Certification Committee
National Clinical Director for Heart Disease,
NHS England & NHS Improvement
Consultant Cardiologist,
James Cook University Hospital, Middlesbrough, UK

Assistant Prof. Dominic Theuns PHD, FEHRA, FESC

Co-chair EHRA Certification Committee
Associate editor Europace
Cardiology Department
Erasmus MC, Rotterdam, the Netherlands

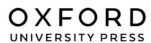

OXFORD
UNIVERSITY PRESS

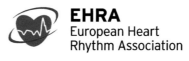

EHRA
European Heart
Rhythm Association

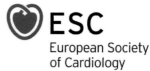

ESC
European Society
of Cardiology

OXFORD
UNIVERSITY PRESS

Great Clarendon Street, Oxford, OX2 6DP,
United Kingdom

Oxford University Press is a department of the University of Oxford.
It furthers the University's objective of excellence in research, scholarship,
and education by publishing worldwide. Oxford is a registered trade mark of
Oxford University Press in the UK and in certain other countries

© European Society of Cardiology 2022

The moral rights of the authors have been asserted

First Edition published in 2015
Second Edition published in 2022

All rights reserved. No part of this publication may be reproduced, stored in
a retrieval system, or transmitted, in any form or by any means, without the
prior permission in writing of Oxford University Press, or as expressly permitted
by law, by licence or under terms agreed with the appropriate reprographics
rights organization. Enquiries concerning reproduction outside the scope of the
above should be sent to the Rights Department, Oxford University Press, at the
address above

You must not circulate this work in any other form
and you must impose this same condition on any acquirer

Published in the United States of America by Oxford University Press
198 Madison Avenue, New York, NY 10016, United States of America

British Library Cataloguing in Publication Data
Data available

Library of Congress Control Number: 2015934017

ISBN 978–0–19–284417–0

DOI: 10.1093/med/9780192844170.001.0001

Printed and bound by CPI Group (UK) Ltd,
Croydon, CR0 4YY

Oxford University Press makes no representation, express or implied, that the
drug dosages in this book are correct. Readers must therefore always check
the product information and clinical procedures with the most up-to-date
published product information and data sheets provided by the manufacturers
and the most recent codes of conduct and safety regulations. The authors and
the publishers do not accept responsibility or legal liability for any errors in the
text or for the misuse or misapplication of material in this work. Except where
otherwise stated, drug dosages and recommendations are for the non-pregnant
adult who is not breast-feeding

Links to third party websites are provided by Oxford in good faith and
for information only. Oxford disclaims any responsibility for the materials
contained in any third party website referenced in this work.

To our teachers, who have shown us that knowledge is a gift that should be shared with generosity, and, most of all, to our loved ones

Endorsement

Professors Burri, Johansen, Linker, and Theuns provide us with yet a new contribution to the European Heart Rhythm Association (EHRA) case-based learning programme.

This new edition provides the reader with 70 cases to troubleshoot pacemaker, implantable cardioverter defibrillator (ICD), and cardiac resynchronization therapy (CRT) device function. It builds on the prior contribution from Burri and colleagues, but this edition provides completely new material, including questions covering conduction system pacing, leadless pacing, and subcutaneous ICDs. This book is the perfect volume for students of our field preparing for certification exams (HRS, EHRA, ABIM). It is a great review for electrophysiology fellows, cardiology fellows, cardiologists, electrophysiologists, nurses, nurse practitioners, and device representatives, engineers, and technicians. I loved challenging myself with these tracings and then checking to make sure my answers were the same as the authors. These books are hard to resist, they are like solving a crossword puzzle. At the end of the day, it is hard to resist this lovely volume; it provides hours of review and testing of one's ability to evaluate device tracings. It is a must have for any student or practitioner of our field. Congratulations to Professors Burri, Johansen, Linker, and Theuns!

Kenneth A. Ellenbogen, MD
Martha M. and Harold W. Kimmerling Professor
Director of Electrophysiology and Pacing
VCU School of Medicine
Richmond, VA, USA

Foreword

I am very pleased to provide a foreword to the second volume of *The EHRA Book of Cardiac Pacing, ICD, and CRT Troubleshooting*. The very successful first volume was published in 2015. Since then, cardiac implantable electronic devices (CIEDs) have seen many improvements, especially with the development of leadless pacing, conduction system pacing, and subcutaneous ICDs. This second volume is authored by four recognized experts in the field of CIEDs, who have been active in the EHRA education or certification committees.

The cases cover a wide range of issues, which are clearly explained. The multiple choice questions are very useful to assess your knowledge on algorithms from the different manufacturers, and also to familiarize yourself with situations you will have to face during follow-up of patients implanted with cardiac devices. Beside the theoretical aspects of CIED function, practise of troubleshooting is essential to acquire the skills for device follow-up. All healthcare providers managing CIEDs (not only physicians but also nurses and technicians) will find great value with this book to increase their knowledge and thus to improve the follow-up of their patients.

This educational book will not only be useful for the preparation of the EHRA Cardiac Pacing certification exam, but will also serve to give better care to device patients.

Professor Christophe Leclercq
EHRA President

Preface

Following the success of the first volume of *The EHRA Book of Pacemaker, ICD, and CRT Troubleshooting* published in 2015, we are very pleased to have been requested to produce a second volume with new cases. This is timely, as device therapy has seen many new developments since the first volume, with the advent of leadless pacing, conduction system pacing, and subcutaneous ICDs, among other novelties. These new technologies are covered here, as are general device troubleshooting issues which were not presented in the first volume.

We have chosen to maintain an identical format for the cases, which are arranged in separate sections on pacing (27 cases), ICDs (23 cases), and CRT (20 cases). Each section is arranged in a logical manner so as to guide the reader to build up on the knowledge gained by the previous cases. As with the first volume, the content will help those planning on sitting the EHRA Cardiac Pacing exam. The level of knowledge may, however, sometimes exceed what is expected of them in the exam. We have gone into more detail regarding specific algorithms of different device manufacturers. It is more important to appreciate the general functionalities of these algorithms, than to memorize their specific details (which can be looked up in different resources), especially as features of these algorithms may evolve over time.

As for the first volume, this book will serve not only to further your technical knowledge, but also to sharpen your skills of observation and reasoning.

We hope you enjoy tackling these tracings!

Haran Burri
Jens Brock Johansen
Nick Linker
Dominic Theuns

Case preparation

All the cases were gathered by the authors from their clinical practice.

Haran Burri: 1–4, 14–25, 28, 31, 33, 38, 40, 43, 47, 50–55, 57, 63, 67, 70.

Jens Brock Johansen: 7, 11, 13, 26, 27, 34–37, 48, 56, 58, 59, 64.

Nick Linker: 6, 9, 12, 29, 30, 32, 39, 41, 42, 68, 69.

Dominic Theuns: 5, 8, 10, 44–46, 49, 60–62, 65, 66.

Acknowledgements

Dr Michael Chapman, for having collected and prepared cases with Professor Nick Linker.

Nurse Lisbeth Skov Nielsen, Odense University Hospital, Denmark, for having helped to collect Dr Johansen's cases.

Dr Tilman Perrin, EHRA Certification Committee member, Solothurn Hospital, Switzerland, for his diligent review of the manuscript.

We are grateful to the following industry employees for having reviewed the cases relating to their devices, and responding to our technical queries:

Abbott: Mr Kunal Chaniary, Mrs Jennifer Rhude, Mr Jordan Vance, Mrs Cortnee Weinrich. *Biotronik*: Mr Jan Iden. *Boston Scientific*: Mr Stefano Acinelli, Mrs Leila Cammoun. Mr Steven Donnelley, Mr Wyatt Stahl. *Medtronic:* Mr Domagoj Elek, Mr Bernd Kaiser, Mrs Tanja Nikolic. *Microport*: Mrs Christelle Deniaud.

Contents

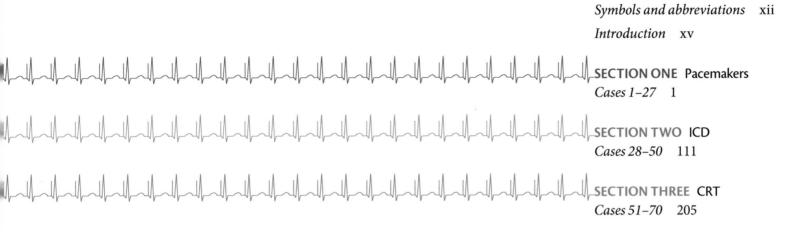

Symbols and abbreviations

=	equal to
≥	equal to or greater than
>	greater than
<	less than
−	minus
%	per cent
+	plus
±	plus or minus
Ab	atrial blanked
AF	atrial fibrillation
AMS	automatic mode switch
AP	atrial pace/pacing
AR	atrial refractory
ARS	atrial refractory sense
AS	atrial sense/sensing
AT	atrial tachycardia
ATDI	atrial tachycardia detection interval
ATP	antitachycardia pacing
AV	atrioventricular
AVB	atrioventricular block
AVI	atrioventricular interval
AVN	atrioventricular node
AVNRT	atrioventricular nodal reciprocating tachycardia
AVRT	atrioventricular reentrant tachycardia
BBB	bundle branch block
bpm	beats per minute
CIED	cardiac implantable electronic device
CRT	cardiac resynchronization therapy
CRT-D	cardiac resynchronization therapy defibrillator
CRT-P	cardiac resynchronization therapy pacemaker
ECG	electrocardiogram
EGM	electrogram
EHRA	European Heart Rhythm Association
EMI	electromagnetic interference
ERI	elective replacement indicator
FARI	filtered atrial rate interval
FFRW	far-field R-wave
HBP	His bundle pacing
ICD	implantable cardioverter defibrillator
LAO	left anterior oblique
LBB	left bundle branch
LBBAP	left bundle branch area pacing
LBBB	left bundle branch block
LOC	loss of capture
LRI	lower rate interval
LV	left ventricular/ventricle
LVEF	left ventricular ejection fraction
LVURI	left ventricular upper rate interval
MAM	manual atrial mechanical
ms	millisecond(s)
MS	mode switch
MTR	maximum tracking rate
Myo	myocardial
NID	number of intervals to detect
ns-HBP	non-selective His bundle pacing
NYHA	New York Heart Association
PAVB	post-atrial ventricular blanking
PLSVC	persistent left superior vena cava

PM	pacemaker	SIR	sensor-indicated rate
PMT	pacemaker-mediated tachycardia	SVC	superior vena cava
PVAB	post-ventricular atrial blanking	SVT	supraventricular tachycardia
PVARP	post-ventricular atrial refractory period	TWOS	T-wave oversensing
PVC	premature ventricular complex	URI	upper rate interval
RA	right atrial/atrium	UTI	upper tracking interval
RBBB	right bundle branch block	UTR	upper tracking rate
RNRVAS	repetitive non-reentrant ventriculoatrial synchrony	VA	ventriculoatrial
RRT	recommended replacement time	VF	ventricular fibrillation
RV	right ventricular/ventricle	VIP	ventricular intrinsic preference algorithm
s	second(s)	VP	ventricular pace/pacing
S-ECG	subcutaneous electrocardiogram	VS	ventricular sense/sensing
s-HBP	selective His bundle pacing	VT	ventricular tachycardia
S-ICD	subcutaneous implantable cardioverter defibrillator	WARAD	window of atrial rate acceleration detection

Introduction

A systematic approach to device electrocardiogram (ECG)/electrogram (EGM) tracings is proposed as a ten-step process, which will allow the reader to troubleshoot cases in a structured manner.

Systematic device electrocardiogram/ electrogram analysis

1 Which ECG leads/EGM channels (chamber, polarity) are displayed, and what is the scale?
2 What is the baseline rhythm?
3 Is there evidence of intrinsic atrial activity, sensing, pacing, and capture?
4 Is there evidence of intrinsic ventricular activity, sensing, pacing, and capture?
5 Are the intervals between the spikes and P/QRS complexes constant?
6 What is the morphology of the paced QRS complex?
7 Evaluation of timing and intervals (AA, VV, AV, VA, etc.).
8 What is the likely pacing mode?
9 Is there evidence of malfunction (undersensing, oversensing, non-pacing, non-capture)?
10 Is there evidence of pseudomalfunction (device algorithm, functional undersensing, etc.)?

Basics of pacemaker troubleshooting

Non-pacing (lack of a spike)

Pseudomalfunction: hysteresis, night rate, device algorithm
Oversensing
Battery/circuit problem
Lead connection problem

Over-pacing (unexpected spike)

Undersensing (atrial or ventricular)
Atrial oversensing (in DDD mode, without modeswitch)
Ventricular oversensing (with noise reversion, or triggered pacing in CRT devices)
Pseudo-dysfunction (device algorithm)
Device dysfunction (e.g. battery depletion)

Non-capture (lack of entrainment of a P-wave or QRS)

Threshold rise: infarction, drugs (flecainide)
Lead problem (insulation defect, fracture, displacement, perforation)
Battery end of life
Programming error

Undersensing

Lead displacement
New bundle branch block, infarction
Premature beat with perpendicular electrogram vector
Programming error
'Physiological undersensing' during refractory period

Oversensing

Ventricular far-field/T-wave/P- or R-wave double counting
Lead problem (fracture, connection problem)
Electromagnetic interference
Myopotentials (pectoral/diaphragmatic)

VVI timing cycles and refractory periods

Timing cycles of the VVI pacing mode are shown in the figure.

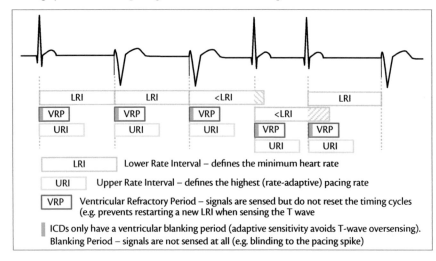

LRI   Lower Rate Interval – defines the minimum heart rate

URI   Upper Rate Interval – defines the highest (rate-adaptive) pacing rate

VRP   Ventricular Refractory Period – signals are sensed but do not reset the timing cycles (e.g. prevents restarting a new LRI when sensing the T wave

ICDs only have a ventricular blanking period (adaptive sensitivity avoids T-wave oversensing). Blanking Period – signals are not sensed at all (e.g. blinding to the pacing spike)

DDD timing cycles and refractory periods

Timing cycles of the DDD pacing mode are shown in the figure.

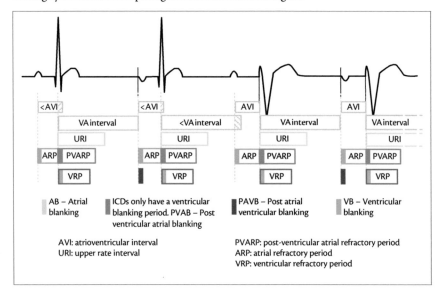

AB – Atrial blanking

ICDs only have a ventricular blanking period. PVAB – Post ventricular atrial blanking

PAVB – Post atrial ventricular blanking

VB – Ventricular blanking

AVI: atrioventricular interval
URI: upper rate interval

PVARP: post-ventricular atrial refractory period
ARP: atrial refractory period
VRP: ventricular refractory period

Summary of DDD timing cycles

A summary of the DDD pacing mode timing cycle triggers and their typical durations is shown in the table.

	AS	AP	VS	VP	Typical duration (ms)
A blanking	✔	✔	✔	✔	50–200
A refractory	✔	✔	✔	✔	120–150 (post AP); 250–400 (post VP)
V blanking		✔	✔	✔	20–50 (post AP); 150–250 (post VP)
V refractory			✔	✔	150–300

Definitions

Blanking: signals are not detected, independent of their amplitude and the programming of sensitivity. Recent devices may, however, sense in the atrial blanking period for the purposes of rhythm diagnosis.

Refractory: signals are detected but will be ignored for pacing cycles (i.e. the timer for next scheduled pace will not be reset) and only used for calculation of rate, detection of tachyarrhythmias, and for mode switching.

Blanking and refractory periods may vary according to

- Device type.
  - ICDs only have a ventricular blanking period, as adaptive sensitivity avoids T-wave oversensing.
    - CRT devices have an interventricular refractory period following a ventricular sensed or paced event to prevent double counting the same ventricular cycle.
- Manufacturer.
- Model.
- Paced or sensed event.
- Programmed pacing polarity.

Main marker channel annotations of different device manufacturers (the list is not exhaustive)

Abbott

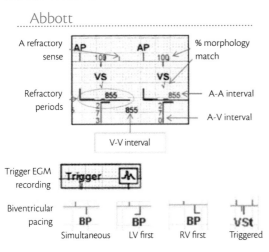

A refractory sense — AP ... AP ... % morphology match
Refractory periods — 855 ... 855 ... A-A interval
855 ... A-V interval
V-V interval

Trigger EGM recording — Trigger

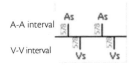

Biventricular pacing — BP (Simultaneous) ... BP (LV first) ... BP (RV first) ... VSt (Triggered)

AMS	Modeswitch
LOC	Loss of capture
VPP	Ventricular backup pacing
–	Interval that is not binned
VS	Binning of interval in sinus zone
T1	Binning of interval in VT1 zone
T2	Binning of interval in VT2 zone
F	Binning of VF interval
F̲	Reconfirmation of VF
SIR	Sensor indicated rate

Microport

A-A interval — As ... As
V-V interval — Vs ... Vs

Ap/A	Atrial pacing
As/P	Atrial sensing
Ar	Atrial refractory sensing
Vs/R	Ventricular sensing
Vp	Ventricular pacing
Vr	Ventricular refractory sensing
bV	Biventricular pacing

Biotronik

As/Ap	Atrial sensing/pacing
Vs/Vp	Ventricular sensing/pacing
LVp/LVs	Left ventricular pacing/sensing
RVp/RVs	Right ventricular pacing/sensing
Ars	Atrial refractory sensing
Ars (FFP)	Ars in far-field protection window
Vrs	Ventricular refractory sensing
Aflut	Atrial flutter detected
Afib	Atrial fibrillation detected
Msw.DDI	Modeswitch to DDI
Det. VF	VF detected
Rdt.	Redetection criteria are fulfilled
1:1	1:1 A:V ratio
	Charging of the capacitors
Term.	Tachycardia episode has terminated
Psh. VVI	Post shock pacing mode is VVI

Boston Scientific

AS	Atrial Sense - After Refractory and AFR window
AS–Hy	Atrial Sense - In Hysteresis Offset
AS–FI	Atrial Sense - In AFR window
(AS)	Atrial Sense - During TARP
[AS]	Atrial Sense - During Blanking
AP	Atrial Pace - Lower Rate
AP↓	Atrial Pace - Rate Smoothing Down
AP↑	Atrial Pace - Rate Smoothing Up
AP–FB	Atrial Pace - Fallback (in ATR)
AP–Hy	Atrial Pace - At Hysteres is Rate
AP–Sr	Atrial Pace - Sensor Rate
AP→	Atrial Pace - Inserted after AFR
AP–Ns	Atrial Pace - Noise (asynchronous pacing)
AP–Tr	Atrial Pace - Trigger Mode
RVS	Right Vent Sense - After Refractory
[RVS]	Right Vent Sense - During Blanking
RVP	Right Vent Pace - Lower Rate or Atrial Tracked
RVP↓	Right Vent Pace - Rate Smoothing Down
RVP↑	Right Vent Pace - Rate Smoothing Up
RVP–FB	Right Vent Pace - Fallback (in ATR)
RVP–Hy	Right Vent Pace - At Hysteresis Rate
RVP–Sr	Right Vent Pace - Sensor Rate
RVP–MT	Right Vent Pace - Atrial Tracked at MTR
RVP–Ns	Right Vent Pace - Noise (asynchronous pacing)
RVP–Tr	Right Vent Pace - Trigger Mode
RVP–VRR	Right Vent Pace - Ventricular Rate Regulation
LVS	Left Vent Sense - After Refractory
[LVS]	Left Vent Sense - During Blanking
LVP	Left Vent Pace - Lower Rate or Atrial Tracked
LVP↓	Left Vent Pace - Rate Smoothing Down
LVP↑	Left Vent Pace - Rate Smoothing Up
LVP–Hy	Left Vent Pace - At Hysteresis Rate
LVP–Sr	Left Vent Pace - Sensor Rate
LVP–MT	Left Vent Pace - Atrial Tracked at MTR
LVP–Ns	Left Vent Pace - Noise (asynchronous pacing)
LVP–Tr	Left Vent Pace - Trigger Mode
LVP–VRR	Left Vent Pace - Ventricular Rate Regulation
Inh–LVP	Left Vent Pace - Inhibited Due to LVPP
PVC	PVC after Refractory
VT–1	VT–1 Zone Sense
VT	VT Zone Sense
VF	VF Zone Sense
AN	Atrial Rate Noise
RVN	Right Ventricular Rate Noise
LVN	Left Ventricular Rate Noise
ATR↓	Atrial Tachycardia Sense - Count Down
ATR↑	Atrial Tachycardia Sense - Count Up
ATR–Dur	ATR Duration Started
ATR–FB	ATR Fallback Started
ATR–End	ATR Fallback Ended
FB	ATR in Progress
RID–TU	Rhythm ID Template Update
RID+	Rhythm ID Correlated
RID–	Rhythm ID Uncorrelated
C––	RhythmMatch^{TM} Correlated without percentage
U––	RhythmMatch^{TM} Uncorrelated without percentage
PVP→	PVARP after PVC
PMT–B	PMT Termination
AF–Rhythm	AFib Rhythm
V–Epsd	Ventricular Tachy Start Episode
V–EpsdEnd	Ventricular Tachy End Episode
V>A	Ventricular Rate Faster than Atrial Rate
AFibV	V AFib Criteria Met
V–Dur	Duration Met
Stb	Stable
Unstb	Unstable
Suddn	Sudden Onset
Gradl	Gradual Onset
V–Detect	Ventricular Detection Met
Chrg	Start/End Charge
Dvrt	Therapy Diverted
Shock	Shock Delivered
SRD	Sustained Rate Duration Expired

Medtronic

AS/AP	Atrial sensing/pacing
AR	Atrial refractory sense
Ab	Atrial event in blanking period
VS/VP	Ventricular sensing pacing
BV	Biventricular pace
VR	Ventricular refractory sense
TS	Sense in (slow) VT zone
T•F	Sense in fast VT zone via VT
TF•	Sense in fast VT zone via VF
FS	Sense in VF zone
TDI	VT detected
TFI	FVT detected
FDI	VF dected
TP	Tachy pace (ATP)
CE	Charge end
CD	Charge delivered

Ventricular safety pacing (V / S)

Triggered biventricular pacing (B / V)

S-ICD

● = Reject
/ = Shock
♥ = End of episode
S = Sensing (normal cycle)
P = Pacing
N = Noise
T = Tachycardia cycle
C = Charge

PACEMAKERS

Cases 1–27

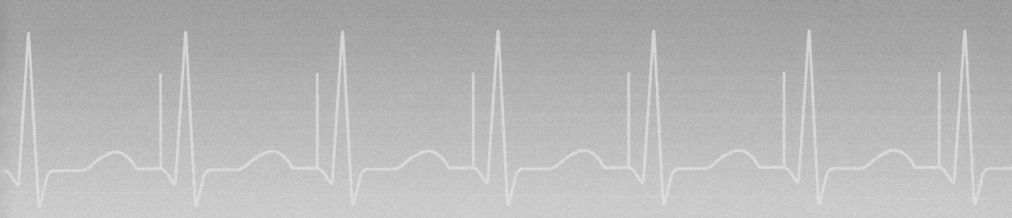

Introduction to the case

A patient was implanted with a DDD pacemaker (PM) for paroxysmal atrioventricular block (AVB). A Holter recording was performed due to palpitations. The tracing corresponding to symptoms is shown in Figure 1.1.

Question

Figure 1.1 Holter recording with tracing during palpitations

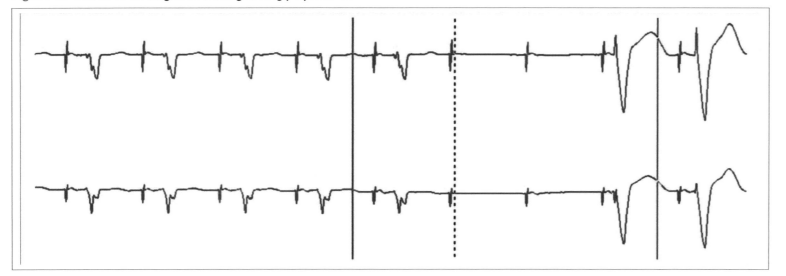

What do you observe?

A Atrial non-capture

B Atrioventricular (AV) hysteresis

C AV management algorithm

D Ventricular non-capture

E Ventricular oversensing

Answer

C AV management algorithm

Figure 1.2 Annotated Holter recording

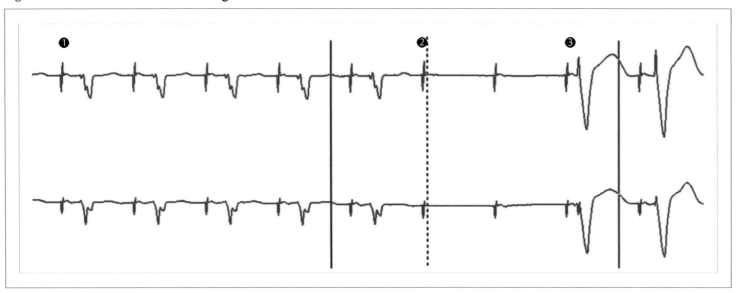

❶ Figure 1.2, the first five cycles correspond to atrial pacing (AP) with intrinsic AV conduction.

❷ Two cycles with AP and capture (note identical timing compared to the previous spikes and the small deflections corresponding to P-waves) and AVB.

❸ The last two cycles correspond to AP and ventricular pacing (VP) (note change in QRS morphology).

Atrial non-capture and atrial hysteresis do not explain the ventricular pause as they would have been followed by VP after the atrioventricular interval (AVI) times out. There is no evidence of ventricular non-capture (i.e. no ventricular spike not followed by a QRS complex).

Ventricular oversensing could explain why the two blocked P-waves are not followed by VP, but does not explain the ventricular pacing of the last two cycles and would have changed the AP–AP intervals.

This behaviour can be explained by the AVB III criterion of the SafeR* algorithm.

Comments

Specific algorithms to minimize ventricular pacing

All major manufacturers have specific algorithms to avoid VP, which are shown in Table 1.1. These algorithms have been shown to effectively reduce unnecessary VP, but some may result in very long PR intervals which can lead to haemodynamic compromise. In rare instances, the pauses resulting from the algorithm may be symptomatic (in the present case, the maximum pause criterion was reduced from 3 s to 2 s, with disappearance of the symptoms). The algorithms are not useful, or should be avoided, in patients with permanent complete AVB, or with a long QT interval (due to a proarrhythmic effect of long–short sequences).

Table 1.1 Features of manufacturer-specific algorithms to avoid ventricular pacing

Algorithm	Primary mode	Switch criterion	Max. pause	2 consecutive blocked P allowed	Very long PR allowed	Recovery check	Switch back criterion
MVP (Medtronic)	AAI(R)/DDD(R)	2/4 Ax without Vs after 420 ms of Ax, or average AVI + 100ms (whichever is longer, but limited to 600ms), AP-VP is delivered with AVI 80 ms# Optional long PR criterion#*	2xLRI, LRI+680 ms#	Yes (at rapid AS rates)	No#*	1,2,4 min... doubling up to **16** h	1 Ax-VS
AAISafeR (Microport)	ADI(R)	AVBIII:2 consecutive Ax without Vs AVBII:3/12 Ax without Vs AVBI: 6 consecutive long AV* Pause: no Vs in 2,3,4s*	2-4s*	Yes	No*	After 100 Vp	12 consecutive Ax-Vs
RythmIQ (Boston Scientific)	AAI(R) + backup VVI 15bpm less than LR	3/11 Vp or slow Vs (= AAI(R) interval +150 ms)	Lower rate — 15 bpm (min 30, max 60)	Yes	Yes	32-1024 cycles (AV hysteresis)	<2/10Vp during AV hysteresis
VP Suppression (Biotronik)	ADI(R)	1,2,3,4* / 8 Ax without Vs, or no Vs for 2 s, or 2 consecutive cycles without Vs. Blocked for 20 h after 15 switches /h.	2 s	Yes	Yes	0 5, 1,2,4 min_ doubling up to 128 min, then 20 h	6 (1-8)* consecutve Vs during 8 cycles of AV hysteresis

Ax, atrial events (for manufacturer abbreviations, see 'Introduction' in the front matter). * Programmable; # feature available in recent models only.

In addition to the algorithms shown in Table 1.1, Abbot, Biotronik, Boston Scientific, Medtronic, and Microport have a programmable positive AV hysteresis algorithm.

Introduction to the case

A patient implanted with a DDD PM for complete AVB was followed-up at the device clinic. He was asymptomatic. A real-time electrogram (EGM) recording is shown in Figure 2.1

.

Question

Figure 2.1 Real-time EGM during follow-up

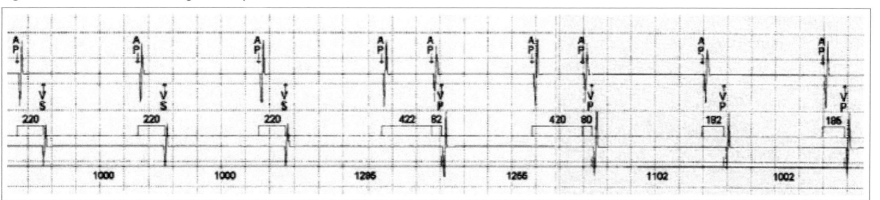

What can be observed?

A Atrial capture threshold algorithm

B Atrial non-capture

C Atrial undersensing

D Managed VP algorithm

E Ventricular safety pacing (VSP)

Answer

D Managed VP algorithm

Figure 2.2 Annotated EGM

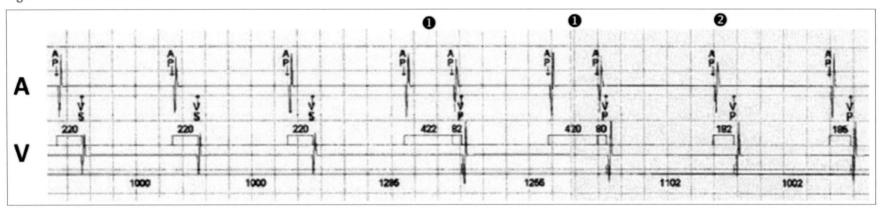

❶ After three AP cycles with intrinsic AV conduction, paroxysmal AVB occurs at the fourth AP event (Figure 2.2). In order to avoid an unduly long pause, VP is delivered. This is preceded 80 ms beforehand by an additional AP event to avoid retrograde conduction and triggering of endless loop tachycardia. This sequence occurs for another cycle.

❷ Because ≥2/4 cycles have demonstrated AVB, the device switches to the DDD mode.

Comments

AAI(R)/DDD(R) mode

This algorithm found in recent Medtronic devices is designed to minimize VP (see Case 1, Table 1.1 for details).

The first version of the algorithm allowed:

- ventricular pauses at 2× the lower rate intervals, with 'long–short' RR sequences (which may be symptomatic or proarrhythmic in certain settings, such as in case of a long QT)

- very long PR intervals with a 'P on T' phenomenon resulting in haemodynamic compromise (simultaneous atrial and ventricular contraction with PM syndrome)—see Volume 1, Case 14).

The revised version of the algorithm, shown here, avoids these issues (the maximum PR interval criterion is programmable).

Introduction to the case

A patient implanted with a dual-chamber PM for sinus dysfunction was followed up. He was asymptomatic. The EGM recording shown in Figure 3.1 was retrieved from the device memory.

Question

Figure 3.1 EGM retrieved from device memory at follow-up

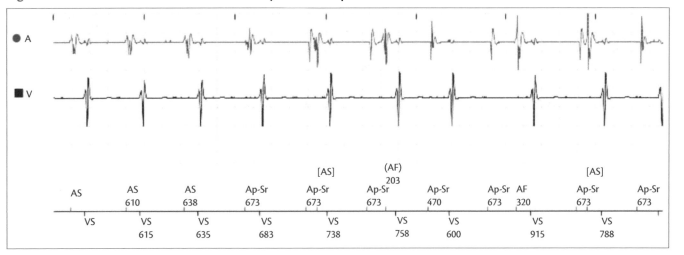

What do you observe?

A Atrial premature beats

B Atrial non-capture

C Far-field R-wave oversensing

D VP avoidance algorithm

E B and D are correct

Answer

E B and D are correct

Figure 3.2 Annotated tracing

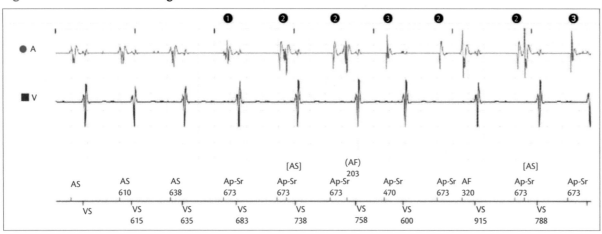

❶ After three cycles of sinus rhythm with intrinsic AV conduction, the sinus rate slows down with AP at the sensor-driven rate (AP–Sr marker) (Figure 3.2). This cycle corresponds to fusion or pseudo-fusion between AP and intrinsic atrial activity (based upon similar morphology compared to the previous beats).

❷ Atrial non-capture, with sensing of the intrinsic rhythm in the atrium corresponding to the [AS] and (AF) markers. Intrinsic AV conduction occurs following the sinus beats ([AS] and (AF) cycles). Small far-field R-waves are visible during all cycles, but are not sensed (no corresponding marker). AP–VS intervals are very long, due to the device functioning in the AAIR/VVI mode (VP avoidance algorithm).

❸ These two cycles have atrial capture, as intrinsic conduction shows reset of ventricular rhythm.

Comments

AAI(R)/VVI mode

This algorithm basically functions similarly to having two devices, the first pacing in AAI(R) at the lower or sensor-driven rate and the second in VVI(R) 15 bpm slower (at a minimum rate of 30 bpm). The episode in this example was retrieved from the device memory due to a switch from AAIR/VVI to DDDR modes due to the slow VS criterion being fulfilled, following atrial non-capture with 3/11 VS intervals being at least 150 ms longer than the AAI(R) intervals (see Case 1, Table 1.1). The EGM with mode switch to DDDR is shown in Figure 3.3.

Figure 3.3 Switch from AAIR/VVI mode to DDDR mode (due to atrial non-capture) indicated by the 'RYTHMIQ' marker. Two slow VS cycles are shown in this strip (920 and 908 ms). The algorithm extends PVARP for one cycle ('PVP→' marker) following switch from a non-tracking to a tracking mode

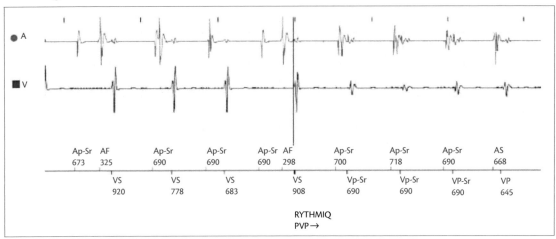

Introduction to the case

A patient implanted with a DDD PM for sinus dysfunction complained of palpitations. A Holter recording was performed. Changes in the rhythm are shown in Figure 4.1, but were unrelated to symptoms.

Question

Figure 4.1 Holter recording with changes in rhythm (recording at 25 mm/s)

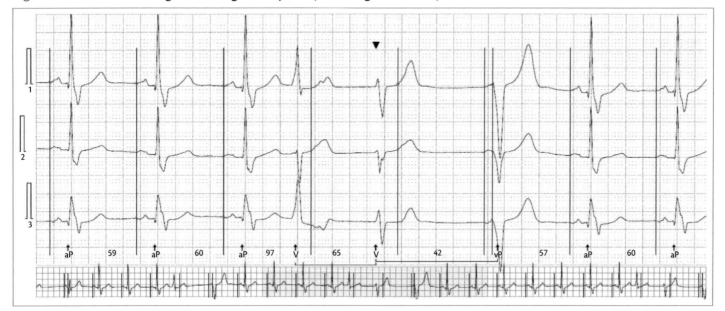

What do you observe?

A Atrial non-capture

B Atrial undersensing

C VP avoidance algorithm

D Ventricular non-capture

E Ventricular undersensing

Answer

C VP avoidance algorithm

Figure 4.2 Annotated Holter recording

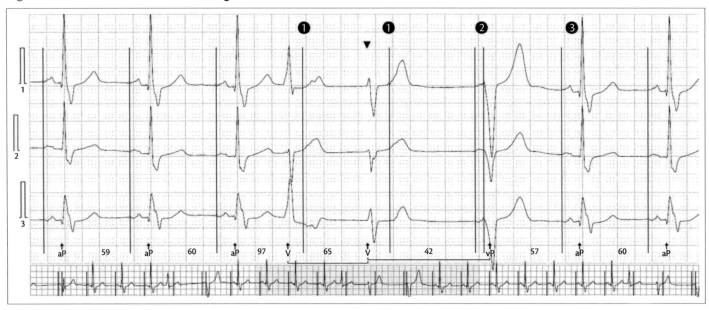

❶ After three cycles of AP and intrinsic conduction, a premature ventricular complex (PVC) occurs (Figure 4.2), but does not disrupt timing of AP (note also the captured P-wave which is clearly visible in the first channel). A second PVC results in the same sequence. The device is functioning in an AAI/VVI mode, whereby AAI pacing is occurring at 60 bpm (the programmed lower rate) with concomitant VVI pacing 15 bpm slower. In the DDD mode, AP would have been reset by ventricular sensing (VS) by triggering a ventriculoatrial (VA) interval. Ventricular undersensing would have resulted in a ventricular spike, which is not visible here.

❷ VVI pacing is occurring at 45 bpm. The VP spike is clearly visible here (and absent on the preceding cycles).

❸ The following beats do not show VP, as the ventricular rate is >45 bpm.

Comments

Algorithms masquerading as device dysfunction

This case illustrates what seems at first glance to be ventricular undersensing, and is in fact a device algorithm designed to minimize VP (see Case 1, Table 1.1). Even though it is difficult (or almost impossible) to memorize the details of all algorithms, the general principles should be known. Furthermore, device dysfunction also results in specific findings which, when absent (such as no VP, ruling out ventricular undersensing in this example), hint towards an algorithm at work. See Figure 4.3.

Figure 4.3 Real-time EGM of a patient with ventricular trigeminy (*) which is interpolated as there is no VA conduction and it does not reset timing of atrial pacing in the AAI/VVI mode (i.e. no VA interval in this mode)

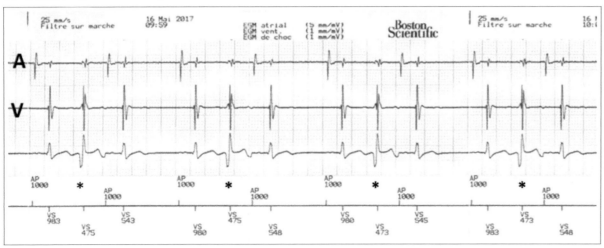

Introduction to the case

A 27-year-old man with congenital heart disease and sick sinus syndrome had been implanted with an epicardial dual-chamber PM, with inactivation of the ventricular lead due to loss of capture (LOC). He was admitted to the emergency room because of palpitations and breathlessness upon exertion. A 12-lead ECG was recorded and is shown in Figure 5.1. Device settings are shown in Table 5.1. A real-time EGM is shown in Figure 5.2.

Figure 5.1 A 12-lead electrocardiogram (ECG) recorded at the emergency room

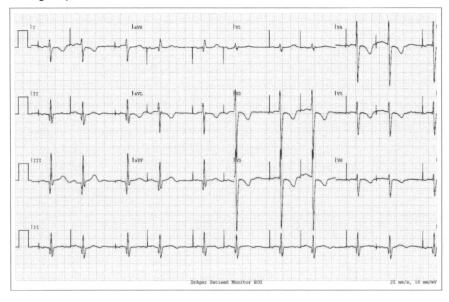

Table 5.1 Device settings

Bradycardia	
Mode	AAIR
Base rate	75 bpm
Pulse amplitude	4 V
Pulse width	1 ms
Sensitivity	Auto
Atrial refractory (AR) period	350 ms

Question

Figure 5.2   Real-time EGM

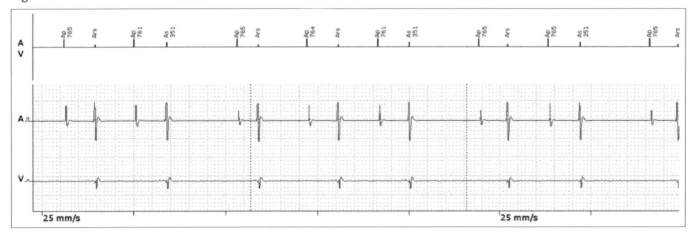

What is your diagnosis?

A Atrial bigeminy

B Atrial non-capture

C AV search hysteresis

D Far-field R-wave (FFRW) oversensing

E Ventricular bigeminy

19

Answer

D Far-field R-wave (FFRW) oversensing

Figure 5.3 Annotated real-time EGM

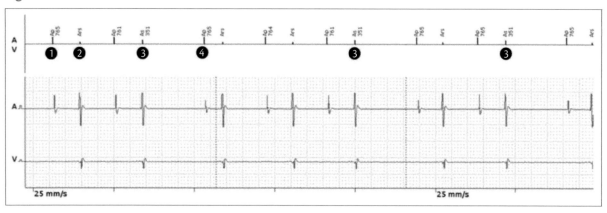

❶ AP with capture and AV conduction with a long PR interval (about 340 ms) is shown in Figure 5.3.

❷ FFRW on the atrial channel, which is synchronous with the signal on the ventricular channel. The FFRW falls in the refractory period (programmed to 350 ms) and is refractory (atrial refractory sense (ARS) marker). It therefore does not reset the lower rate interval (LRI) timer and the following AP occurs at 761 ms.

❸ AV conduction shows a Wenckebach pattern with prolongation of the PR interval. The FFRW is now sensed just beyond the refractory period, at 351 ms, and resets the LRI timer.

❹ AP occurs at 765 + 351 = 1116 ms (54 bpm) from the last paced event. Note that the PR interval here is shortened due to recovery of atrioventricular nodal (AVN) conduction after the pause.

Comments

Caveats of AAIR pacing

Since the results of the DANPACE trial, AAIR pacing is rarely used due to a higher incidence of atrial fibrillation (AF) and system revision compared to DDDR pacing.[1] This pacing modality may, however, sometimes be programmed in patients with isolated sinus node dysfunction in case of issues with ventricular pacing, as in the present case. FFRW oversensing is a major issue and should be avoided by programming long refractory periods which should take into account AV conduction. Another option would be to reduce atrial sensitivity, which, however, would probably not be useful in the present case due to the high amplitude of the FFRW.

In the present case, therapeutic options would be to prolong the AR period, or programme the device to an ADIR (or if unavailable, to a DDIR mode with subthreshold ventricular output) in order to benefit from the post-ventricular atrial blanking (PVAB). However, this patient had symptoms at exercise which would no doubt have persisted despite these measures in the absence of effective VP, due to Wenckebach AV block. System revision will ultimately be necessary, also in view of the high pacing output from the atrial lead which will result in premature battery depletion in this young patient.

Reference

1. Nielsen JC, Thomsen PEB, Højberg S, et al. A comparison of single-lead atrial pacing with dual-chamber pacing in sick sinus syndrome. *Eur Heart J* 2011; **32**: 686–696.

Introduction to the case

A 64-year-old woman attended clinic following several episodes of short-lived, unprovoked palpitations. These had occurred several times per week since her device was implanted. She had a DDD PM implanted 3 months earlier due to syncope associated with sinus pauses on an implantable loop recorder. Her device EGM is shown in Figure 6.1

.

Question

Figure 6.1   EGM retrieved from the PM memory

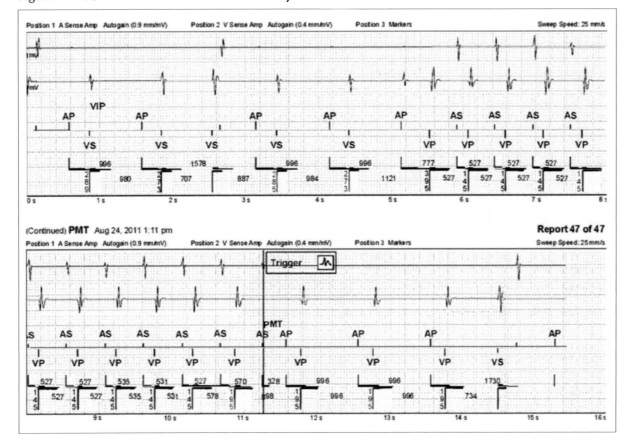

By what mechanism has this pacemaker-mediated tachycardia (PMT) occurred?

A   An atrial premature complex

B   A PVC falling within the PVAB

C   Atrial LOC

D   AV hysteresis

E   Ventricular oversensing

Answer

D AV hysteresis

Figure 6.2 Annotated EGM

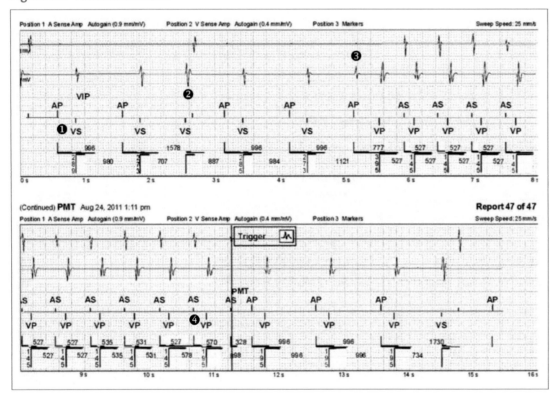

❶ Ventricular intrinsic preference (VIP) pacing (Figure 6.2): the VIP marker indicates that the current paced AV delay is longer than programmed. This is due to AV hysteresis whereby the device periodically extends the AV delay beyond programmed (up to a maximum limit) to allow for intrinsic AV conduction to occur where possible. The cycles are AP with intrinsic ventricular conduction. Note the low signal amplitude on the atrial channel due to damping on this channel after AP (and masquerading as atrial non-capture).

❷ An isolated PVC. Note the P wave occurring shortly afterwards. This begins with a Q wave and is of different morphology to those retrograde P waves seen during the PMT and likely represents normal sinus rhythm rather than retrograde VA conduction (which is also suggested by the short VA interval).

❸ A PVC falls at the same time as AP and is blanked in the PAVB (and not the PVAB, as suggested in option B). The AV timer is triggered, with a prolonged AV delay (395 ms) due to VIP. Due to this long AV delay, the AVN is no longer refractory and retrograde conduction occurs, triggering endless loop tachycardia.

❹ After ten repetitive AS–VP events at/near the maximum track rate, a PMT algorithm activates. In this device, the AV delay is increased by 50 ms (from 145 to 195 ms). The AA delay also prolongs (by 43 ms, from 522 ms to 570 ms) indicating the atria are being driven by the ventricles, confirming PMT. The device terminates this event by a further AP beat, rendering the AVN refractory to VA conduction.

Comments

Endless loop tachycardia recognition algorithms

PMTs are usually suspected by devices when AS–VP occurs at rates close to the programmed upper rate. Algorithms then confirm the mechanism by either extending/shortening the AV interval and measuring the resulting VA interval, or by extending the post-ventricular atrial refractory period (PVARP) (Table 6.1).

Table 6.1 Endless loop tachycardia recognition algorithms of different manufacturers

Algorithm	Activation	Intervention
Abbott	8 consecutive VP–AS cycles > PMT detect rate	*Evaluation*: AVI altered for 1 cycle: shortened by 50 ms (if AS–VP >100 ms); extended by 50 ms (if AS–VP <100 ms) *Confirmation*: if VP–AS within 16 ms of ΔAVI, endless loop tachycardia is confirmed *Intervention*: VP suspended for 1 cycle; AP delivered 330 ms after detected retrograde P wave
Biotronik	8 successive VP–AS cycles < programmable VA criterion, *and* variation <25 ms	*Evaluation*: AVI or MTR is modified for 1 cycle *Confirmation*: if VP–AS stable, PMT confirmed *Intervention*: PVARP extended to VA interval + 50 ms
Boston Scientific	16 consecutive AS–VP cycles at MTR, and variation in VA intervals by <32 ms	PVARP extended to 500 ms for 1 cycle
Medtronic	8 consecutive VP–AS cycles <400 ms	*Detection phase* followed by *confirmation phase* with adjustment of timing of VP. If VP timing affects timing of AS for 3 consecutive groups of VP–AS intervals, a PMT is confirmed. PVARP extended to 400 ms for 1 cycle on 9th VP
Microport	8 consecutive VP–AS cycles ≤470 ms and stable (with ≤30 ms variation)	*Evaluation*: shortening of AV interval by 50 or 65 ms depending on variability of VA is less or greater than 15 ms respectively. If this violates the upper pacing rate, the AV interval is lengthened *Confirmation*: VA interval is stable within 15 ms *Intervention*: PVARP extended to 500 ms

MTR, maximum tracking rate.

Introduction to the case

A child with an epicardial DDD PM system due to a third-degree AVB is seen at follow-up.

The device parameters are shown in Figure 7.1, and an EGM retrieved from the device memory is displayed in Figure 7.2.

Figure 7.1 Device parameters

ST. JUDE MEDICAL — **Assurity™ + DR 2260 Pacemaker** 4488409 — **Jan 25, 2019** **10:00 am** Archive

Parameters

Page 1 of 2

Patient | **Indications for Implant**
Date of Birth
EF % Unknown

Device	**Manufacturer**	**Model**	**Serial**	**Implant Date**
Pacemaker	St. Jude Medical	Assurity™ + DR 2260	4488409	Nov 25, 2014
A Lead				
V Lead				

Device cybersecurity upgrade is available

Basic Operation	
Mode	DDD
V. Triggering	Off
Magnet Response	Battery Test
V. Noise Reversion Mode	DOO
Sensor	Off

Rates	
Base Rate	60 bpm
Rest Rate	Off
Max Track Rate	180 bpm
Hysteresis Rate	Off
2:1 Block Rate	236 bpm

Delays	
Paced AV Delay	160 ms
Sensed AV Delay	130 ms
Rate Responsive AV Delay	Medium
Shortest AV Delay	80 ms
Ventricular Intrinsic Preference (VIP™)	Off
Negative AV Hysteresis/Search	Off

Refractories & Blanking	
PVARP	300 ms
Post-Vent. Atrial Blanking	150 ms
Rate Responsive PVARP/V Ref	High
Shortest PVARP/V Ref	175 ms
A/V Pace Refractory	190/250 ms
A/V Sense Refractory	93/250 ms
Ventricular Blanking	44 ms
Ventricular Safety Standby	On
PVC Response	Off
PMT Response	Atrial Pace
PMT Detection Rate	130 bpm

AT/AF Detection & Response	
Auto Mode Switch	VVI
A. Tachycardia Detection Rate	225 bpm
AMS Base Rate	80 bpm
AF Suppression™	Off

Capture & Sense	**A**	**V**
V. AutoCapture		Off
Pulse Amplitude	2.5 V	2.5 V
Pulse Width	0.4 ms	1.0 ms
AutoSense	Off	Off
Sensitivity (Safety Margin)	0.75 mV (4.5:1)	1.0 mV

Leads	**A**	**V**
Lead Type	Unipolar	Bipolar
Pulse Configuration	Unipolar	Bipolar
Sense Configuration	Unipolar Tip	Bipolar
Lead Monitoring	Monitor	Monitor
Lower Limit	200 Ω	200 Ω
Upper Limit	2,000 Ω	2,000 Ω

Congestion Monitoring	
Congestion Monitoring	Off

Last Programmed: Jan 5, 2018 11:58 am
Parameters that are "n/a" are not shown

Bold values were changed this session (See Wrap-up™ Overview report for details)

▸ Manual-programmed
↳ Auto-programmed
Ⓐ Automatic

Assurity™ + DR 2260 Pacemaker (4488409 pr14.07.75)
Merlin™ PCS (#14243 3330 v24.2.2 rev 1)

Parameters Page 1 of 2
Jan 25, 2019 10:00 am

Question

Figure 7.2 EGM retrieved from the device memory

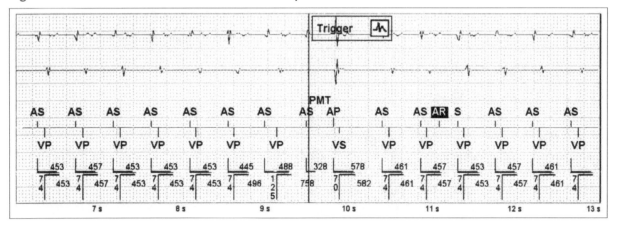

What do you observe?

A 2:1 Wenckebach block

B Atrial undersensing

C Correct PMT diagnosis

D Incorrect PMT diagnosis

E Negative hysteresis

Answer

D Incorrect PMT diagnosis

Figure 7.3 Annotated EGM

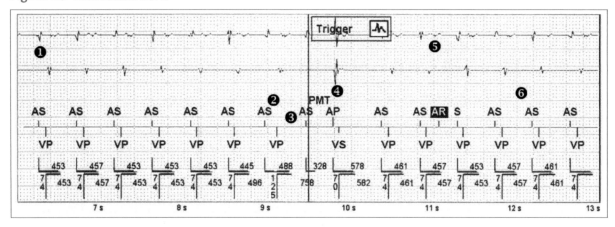

❶ Sinus tachycardia above programmed PMT detection rate (130 bpm) (Figure 7.3).

❷ The device extends the AVI by 50 ms as a first step to test for PMT (had the AV interval been ≥100 ms, the device would have shortened the AVI by 50 ms).

❸ There is a coincidental prolongation of the AS–AS interval by 43 ms (with little change in the VA interval), which is interpreted by the device as proof that this is a retrograde atrial event, and PMT is diagnosed. The device delivers AP 330 ms after the last AS event to regain AV synchrony.

❹ PVC occurring almost simultaneously with AP and sensed in the ventricular channel after 70 ms. Ventricular safety pacing is not delivered, as the window is 64 ms in this device (other manufacturers have windows of >100 ms and would have delivered VP).

❺ Intermittent FFRW oversensing (AR marker).

❻ The atrial rate does not change significantly compared to before PMT intervention. This makes endless loop tachycardia very unlikely.

Comments

Endless loop tachycardia detection and termination algorithms

Endless loop tachycardia is one of the aetiologies of PMT (other examples being sensor-driven tachycardia, tracking of supraventricular arrhythmias due to inactivation of mode switch, and runaway pacemaker). Devices usually suspect endless loop tachycardia when the atrial rate is at the MTR or if the VA interval is below a certain value. In Abbott devices (such as the one in the present case), the programmable 'PMT detection rate' is by default programmed equal to MTR but was for an unknown reason programmed lower in this patient. Once eight consecutive VP-AS cycles exceed the PMT detection rate, this algorithm identifies retrograde conduction by measuring a constant VA interval after having varied the AV interval (Figure 7.4).

Figure 7.4 Abbott algorithm for identifying endless loop tachycardia. The AS–VP interval is either lengthened (if it is <100 ms, as in Figures 7.2 and 7.3) or shortened (if it is ≥100 ms, as depicted here). Supraventricular tachycardia (SVT) or endless loop tachycardia is diagnosed based upon the change or maintenance of the VA interval respectively

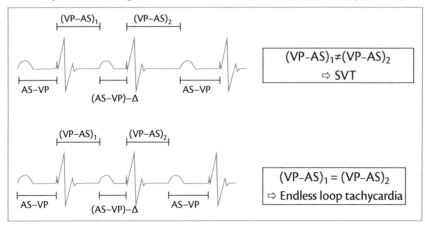

Other devices check for endless loop tachycardia when the AS–VP rate is at the MTR or if the VA interval is below a certain value. Once identified, endless loop tachycardia is terminated by withholding VP for one cycle (as in the present case) or by extending the PVARP by a cycle, which allows the retrograde P wave to be refractory and not tracked (see Case 6, Table 6.1).

Introduction to the case

A patient implanted with a dual-chamber PM for brady–tachy syndrome was seen at follow-up. He had no complaints. The episode shown in Figure 8.1 was retrieved from the device memory.

Question

Figure 8.1 Automatic mode switch episode retrieved from the device memory

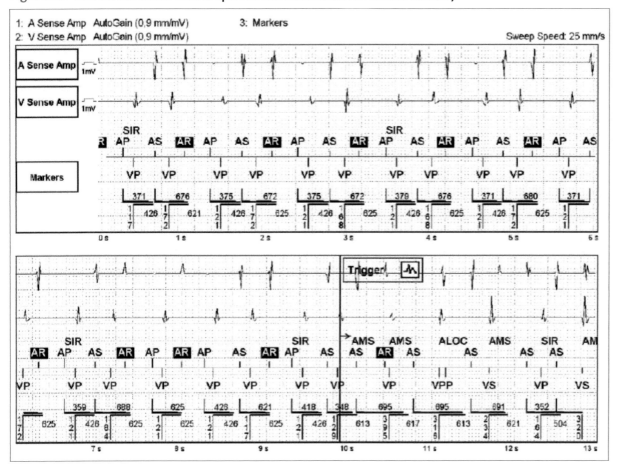

What is the cause for the mode switch?

A Atrial arrhythmia

B Endless loop tachycardia

C FFRW oversensing

D Repetitive non-reentrant ventriculoatrial synchrony (RNRVAS)

E None of the above

Answer

A Atrial arrhythmia

Figure 8.2 Annotated tracing

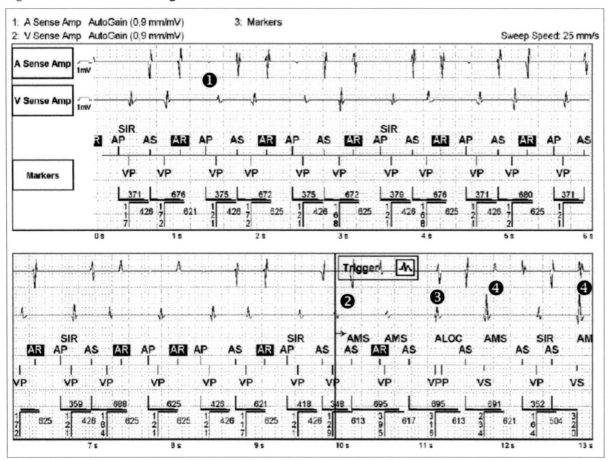

❶ Atrial activity appears to be bigeminal (Figure 8.2). However, signal damping during AP cycles at sensor-indicated rate (SIR) masks possible simultaneous intrinsic atrial activity.

❷ Automatic mode switch (AMS) criteria are met, with DDIR pacing. Absence of AP cycles reveals that atrial tachyarrhythmia is continuous, and not bigeminal (with intrinsic signals which were previously masked during AP).

❸ LOC in the ventricular channel probably results from pseudo-fusion due to intrinsic AV conduction (note presence of subsequent VS cycles). An atrial potential is visible but falls in the PVAB (no marker visible on the marker channel). The 'ALOC' marker is a printing overlap between 'AMS' and 'LOC'.

❹ Atrial activity falling in the PVAB.

Comments

Mode switching due to atrial tachyarrhythmias

Mode switching should be activated in all dual/triple-chamber devices, to avoid tracking of atrial tachyarrhythmias which results in rapid VP and possible deleterious effects on cardiac function. A summary of the mode switching algorithms is shown in Table 8.1.

Table 8.1 Mode switch algorithms of different device manufacturers

	Abbott	Biotronik	Boston Scientific	Medtronic	Microport
Entry criteria	FARI < ATDI AA < FARI: $FARI_{new} = FARI_{old} - 39$ ms AA > FARI: $FARI_{new} = FARI_{old} + 23$ ms Recent devices: AR–AP intervals not counted	X/8 intervals (default 5/8) < mode switch interval	1–8 cycles (with count +1 above and −1 below the ATR rate). All atrial events except for Ab cycles or in noise windows are counted. Once entry count is met, a programmable duration criterion (ATR-Dur) is triggered	3 VV intervals with ≥2 intervening atrial events AND median of last 12 A–A intervals < ATR	WARAD refractory period based on acceleration of previous As–As interval (75% if >80 bpm, 62.5% if <80 bpm). Suspicion and confirmation phases
Detect rate	Programmable	Programmable	Programmable	Programmable	Non-programmable (dependent on WARAD; mode switch may occur below MTR)
Fallback pacing mode*	DDI(R), DDT(R), off	DDI(R) or VDI(R)	VDI(R) or DDI(R)	DDIR (or VDIR if programmed to VDD)	DDI(R)
Lower rate in mode switch	Separately programmable	Separately programmable	Separately programmable	Not programmable (= base/sensor rate)	Not programmable (= base/sensor rate)
Transition of ventricular rate	Sudden	Gradual	Gradual (programmable)	Gradual	Gradual
Exit criteria	FARI > MTR interval or SIR interval, whichever is longer	X/8 intervals (default 5/8) > mode switch interval	1–8 exit counter below ATR trigger rate	7 A–A longer than UTI, or 5 consecutive AP	Atrial and ventricular rates are both <107 bpm. Confirmation phase = 24 cycles after arrhythmia end and no PAC over the last 12 cycles
Atrial flutter detection		2:1 lock-in management	Atrial flutter response (resetting of refractory window corresponding to the ATR interval following sensing in PVARP)	Blanked flutter search	

Ab, atrial blanked; AFR, atrial flutter response; AMR, automatic mode switch; AR, atrial refractory; ATDI, atrial tachycardia detection interval; ATR, atrial tachycardia response; FARI, filtered atrial rate interval; MTR, maximum tracking rate; SIR, sensor indicated rate UTI, upper tracking interval; WARAD, window of atrial rate acceleration detection.

* In cardiac resynchronization therapy (CRT) devices, VVT mode may also be triggered as a secondary mode during mode switch (up to a programmable upper ventricular rate), to deliver biventricular or left ventricular (LV) pacing during conducted atrial arrhythmias.

Introduction to the case

A 73-year-old man had been implanted with a DDD PM for brady–tachy syndrome. He attended the device clinic, reporting several episodes of unprovoked palpitations. Device parameters are shown in Table 9.1. An EGM of a mode switch episode is shown in Figure 9.1.

Table 9.1 Device parameters

Mode	DDDR
Base rate	60 bpm
Upper tracking rate (UTR)	110 bpm
Maximum sensor rate	110 bpm
Paced AV delay	200 ms
Sensed AV delay	180 ms
PVARP	275 ms
PVAB	60 ms
PMT detection rate	110 bpm
Atrial tachycardia (AT) detection rate	180 bpm
Automatic mode switch base rate	60 bpm

Question

Figure 9.1 EGM of stored episode

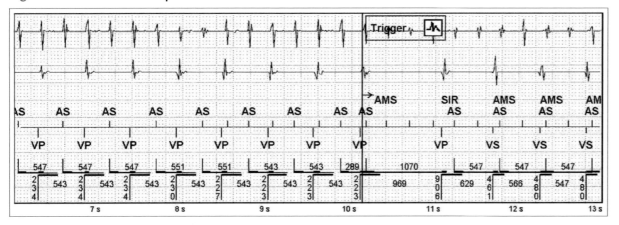

What problem do you observe?

A Atrial flutter lock-in

B Endless loop tachycardia

C FFRW oversensing

D Inappropriate mode switching

E Upper rate behaviour

Answer

A Atrial flutter lock-in

Figure 9.2 Annotated EGM

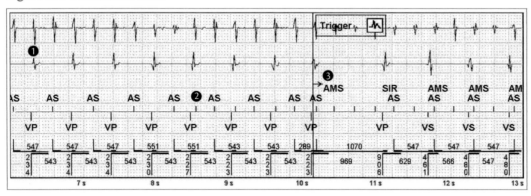

The 2:1 blanked flutter was revealed by the mode switch episode (and would otherwise have not been recorded) (Figure 9.2).

❶ Alternate flutter waves are blanked in the PVAB, with tracking of the atrial events. The AV delay is extended in order not to violate the programmed MTR of 110 bpm (cycle length of 545 ms). Endless loop tachycardia would have a 1:1 AV ratio.

❷ The previously blanked atrial signals are now sensed in the PVARP, due to slightly delayed sensing (short vertical bars without a marker annotation).

❸ Once the mode switching criteria are fulfilled, appropriate mode switching is triggered. Potentials in the atrial channel are unaffected by the absence of VP, so this cannot be FFRW oversensing. In Abbott devices, there is no PVARP during mode switch (only PVAB), explaining the AS events. Subsequent atrial sensing will be labelled as refractory ('|' markers) until a VP/VS event occurs.

Comments

Atrial flutter lock-in/blanked flutter

Atrial flutter lock-in occurs when alternate flutter waves are blanked, preventing mode switching with 2:1 tracking of atrial activity. The issue is outlined in Box 9.1.

Figure 9.3 Graphic depiction of 2:1 lock-in flutter/blanked flutter illustrating requirement of AVI+PVAB>flutter interval. **1.** Long AVI. Atrial flutter equalling half the upper tracking rate starts before the upper tracking rate interval elapses, with extension of the AVI, which is then maintained at this extended value during 2:1 locked-in flutter. **2.** Long programmed PVAB. Every second atrial flutter event falls in the PVAB.

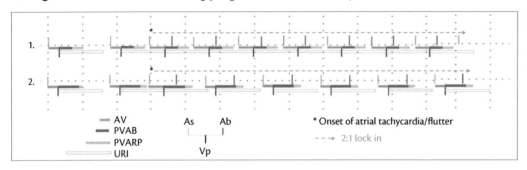

Box 9.1 Synopsis of 2:1 flutter lock-in/blanked flutter

Prerequisites

- AVI + PVAB > atrial flutter cycle length.
- AT detection rate > half the flutter rate (otherwise mode switch occurs with consecutive flutter cycles which fall outside the PVAB).
- MTR ≥ half the flutter rate.

Initiation and maintenance

- Every second atrial cycle falls in the PVAB.

Termination

- Consecutive atrial cycles fall out of the PVAB with AS–AR sequence:
  - Slowing of flutter and refractory sensing in the PVARP.
  - Acceleration of flutter and refractory sensing in the AVI.
- Device algorithm (PVARP or AVI extension).

Predisposing factors

- Long PVAB.
- High UTR.
- High AT detection rate.
- Long AVI (predisposes the following atrial cycle to fall in the PVAB).

Protecting factors

- Short PVAB (but predisposes to FFRW oversensing).
- AV delay programmed longer than tachycardia cycle length (following atrial cycle is sensed as refractory).
- Short AVI/rate adaptive AVI (allows the following atrial cycle to be sensed in the PVARP).
- Low AT detection rate (but may result in mode switch during sinus rhythm).
- Specific device algorithms.

Introduction to the case

A 45-year-old man with a total AVB after a Bentall procedure had been implanted with a dual-chamber PM. During follow-up, he experienced dizzy spells during moderate exercise. The device settings are shown in Table 10.1. Real-time recording during a bicycle exercise test is shown in Figure 10.1.

Table 10.1 Device settings

Bradycardia		
Mode	DDD	
Base rate	60 bpm	
Upper track rate	160 bpm	
AV delay	Paced	Sensed
At 60 bpm	180 ms	135 ms
At 140 bpm	140 ms	95 ms
PVARP	225 ms	
PMT protection	On	
VA criterion	350 ms	
Mode switch rate	180 bpm	

Question

Figure 10.1 Real-time EGM recorded during a bicycle exercise test

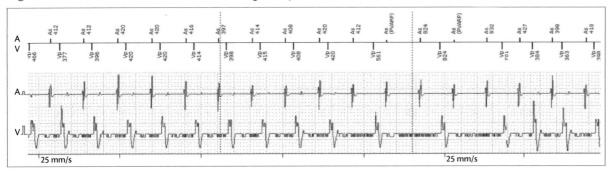

What is your diagnosis?

A 2:1 lock-in protection algorithm

B Atrial oversensing

C Endless loop tachycardia algorithm

D Mode switch

E Upper rate behaviour

Answer

A 2:1 lock-in protection algorithm

Figure 10.2 Annotated real-time EGM recorded during a bicycle exercise test

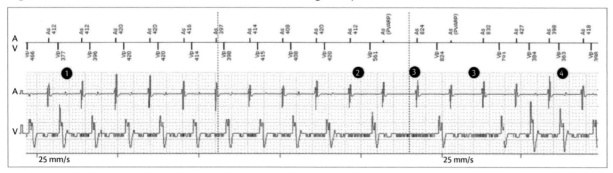

❶ The atrial EGM (Figure 10.2) shows high- and low-amplitude signals. The high-amplitude signals represent intrinsic atrial events at a rate of 144 bpm (which is well below the UTR), and the low-amplitude signals represent FFRWs, which are not sensed by the device (no markers on the atrial channel).

❷ Sudden prolongation of AVI (by the value of the programmed PVAB, which is 150 ms by default) is triggered by the 2:1 protection algorithm, which causes a transient drop in ventricular rate. Wenckebach or upper rate behaviour can be ruled out, as the previous intervals demonstrate a stable AV delay. The AVI remains prolonged over the following cycles, which would be unusual for an endless loop tachycardia detection algorithm (which usually changes settings for one cycle only).

❸ Sinus tachycardia continues, with two atrial events detected in one VP–VP interval. One atrial event is detected in the PVARP and the other atrial event is tracked with a prolonged AVI. However, the atrial rate is below the mode switch rate.

❹ 1:1 atrial tracking is restored by progressively decreasing the AV delay to the programmed value (over a maximum of four cardiac cycles). This is also not typical of an endless loop tachycardia detection algorithm.

Comments

2:1 lock-in protection algorithm

Atrial tachyarrhythmias may lead to 2:1 lock-in when every second atrial event falls in the PVAB, with tracking of every second atrial cycle and rapid VP (see Case 9). Biotronik devices have an algorithm which prolongs the AVI by the programmed PVAB (otherwise known as the 'far-field protection window' of 150 ms by default, programmable up to 220 ms) in order to uncover blanked atrial activity. If atrial activity faster than the mode switch rate is detected in the extended AVI, 2:1 lock-in is confirmed (Figure 10.3). This algorithm can be inactivated if preferred.

Figure 10.3 Example of 2:1 lock-in flutter with every second flutter wave falling in the PVAB, denoted by the ARS (FFP) marker. The algorithm suddenly prolongs the AVI (*), unmasking the flutter, and leading to mode switch. Had the ARS (FFP) events been simply due to far-field R-waves, extension of the AVI would have been accompanied by a fixed VP–ARS (FFP) sequence

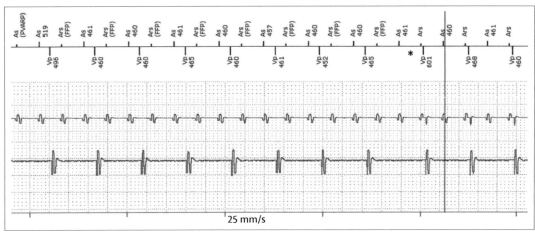

25 mm/s

Introduction to the case

A patient had undergone aortic valve replacement and was equipped with temporary epicardial pacing. Telemetry ECG strips recorded on the ward 5 days after surgery are shown in Figure 11.1.

Question

Figure 11.1 Telemetry rhythm strips (tracings are consecutive)

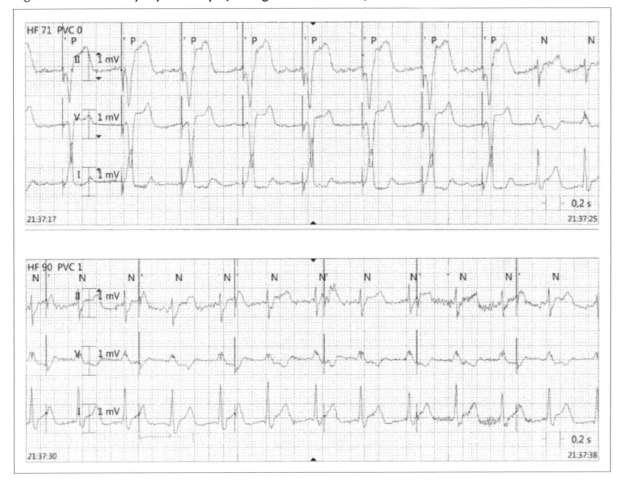

Which of the following best describes the rhythm strips?

A Atrial undersensing

B Intermittent loss of atrial capture

C Intermittent loss of ventricular capture

D Normal DDD pacing

E Ventricular undersensing

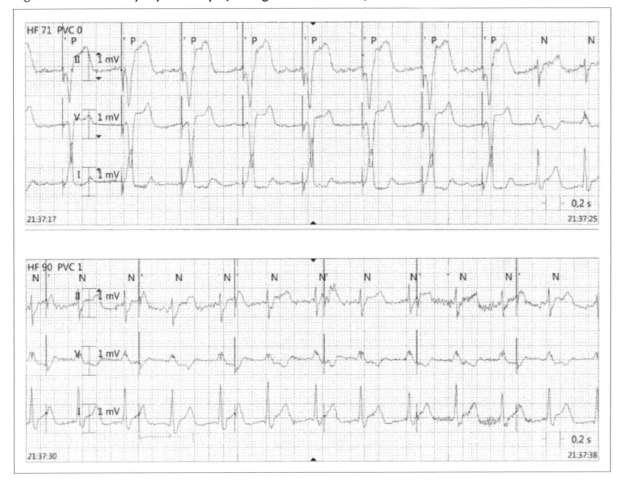

Answer

E Ventricular undersensing

Figure 11.2 Annotated telemetry rhythm strips

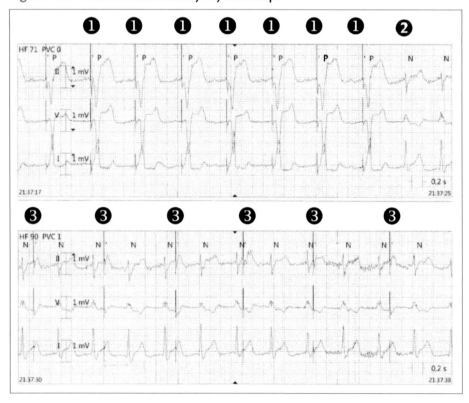

The original temporary epicardial pacemaker was a DDD system, but due to poor function of the atrial lead, the atrial channel had been disabled, and pacing had been programmed to VVI (Figure 11.2).

❶ VP at programmed lower rate (around 70 bpm). Every paced cycle is captured.

❷ Intrinsic heart rate increases slightly above programmed lower rate and is appropriately sensed (no pacing spike is visible).

❸ Intermittent undersensing of every second beat of the intrinsic rhythm, which is faster than the programmed lower rate. This causes VP to be delivered close to the vulnerable phase of the QRS complex.

Comments

Proarrhythmia due to undersensing

Ventricular undersensing with asynchronous pacing in the vulnerable period in this patient ultimately resulted in ventricular fibrillation (VF) (Figure 11.3). The patient was successfully resuscitated.

Figure 11.3 Ventricular undersensing with asynchronous pacing on the ascending limb of the T-wave in the vulnerable period, resulting in VF. Note intermittent undersensing of VF with delivery of pacing spikes

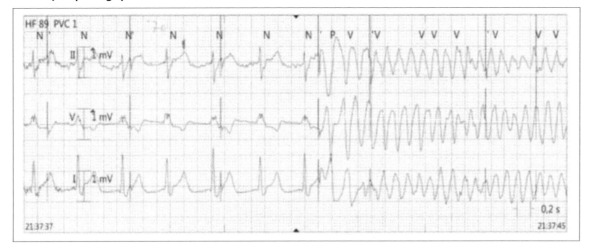

Due to instability or to pericardial effusion/inflammation, temporary epicardial wires are prone to dysfunction, and should be checked on a daily basis.

Back in the era of transtelephonic device follow-ups, proarrhythmia was seldom reported, despite temporary asynchronous pacing. Nevertheless, it is recommended to have an external defibrillator for in-office follow-ups as arrhythmias may exceptionally be triggered from asynchronous pacing due to magnet response during application of the telemetry head or during lead testing. The external defibrillator should also be capable of delivering transcutaneous pacing, as wireless telemetry may drain a battery at end of life and result in LOC.

Introduction to the case

A 45-year-old man presented to the emergency room with several episodes of presyncope. The majority of these were unprovoked episodes, but he was able to reproduce his symptoms by leaning forwards. He had a dual-chamber PM implanted 9 years previously following iatrogenic AVB during ablation for atrioventricular nodal reentrant tachycardia (AVNRT). He was otherwise fit and well. His EGM is shown in Figure 12.1.

Question

Figure 12.1 EGM recorded while leaning forwards

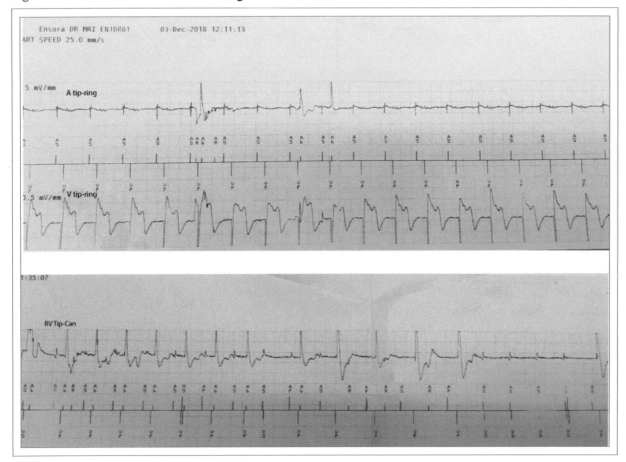

What problem best describes the findings in the EGM?

A Atrial and ventricular lead mismatch in device header

B Atrial lead displacement into ventricle

C Insulation breach on atrial and ventricular leads

D Ventricular lead displacement into atria

E Ventricular lead fracture

Answer

C Insulation breach on atrial and ventricular leads

Figure 12.2 Annotated EGM

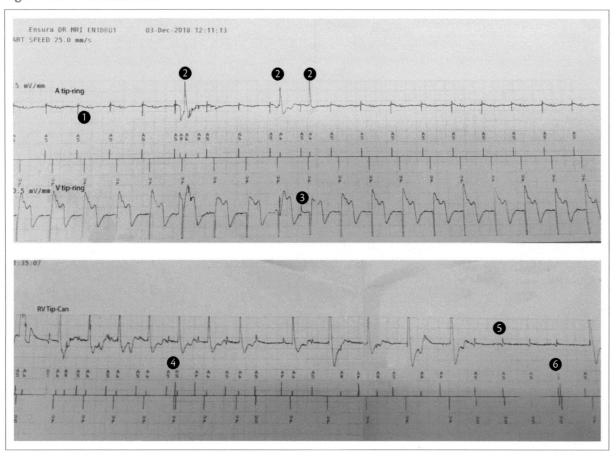

❶ Atrial sensed (AS) signals measuring approximately 2–2.5 mV with small FFRW which are not sensed (no Ab marker) (Figure 12.2).

❷ Intermittent noise on atrial channel (AR) with large, RV pacing spike seen intermittently on atrial channel and falling within PVAB period (Ab).

❸ P-wave seen intermittently on ventricular channel, which is not sensed.

❹ Mode switch ('MS' marker) to DDIR mode. Note the subsequent paced AV delays which are fixed, and sensed AV delays which are variable, a hallmark of DDI(R) timing.

❺ P-wave oversensing in the ventricular channel, leading to inhibition of pacing, with transient asystole.

❻ The device returns to DDD mode after AS–VS sequences.

Comments

Insulation breach

Lead insulation breach is a rare complication of PM implantation, occurring in <1% of pacing leads. It typically occurs due to subclavian crush but can occur at any point along the length of the lead. Most pacing leads have a coaxial design with an innermost tip conductor surrounded by an outer ring conductor, which are separated by a layer of insulation (with additional outer insulation). Insulation breach is characterized by a drop in lead impedance although this may not always be apparent due to the intermittent nature of impedance checks. If lead impedance drops, batteries become susceptible to current drain, and capture thresholds may increase due to current dispersion. Furthermore, oversensing of myopotentials may occur. This is more common in bipolar sensing/pacing configuration, as this relies on the ring conductor which is more exposed to external wear than the inner tip conductor. When insulation breach occurs from lead–lead interaction, cross-sensing may occur, as in the present example.

Temporary management could be to programme pacing and sensing configuration to unipolar and ruling out oversensing, or programming in DOO/VOO mode, while awaiting lead revision.

Introduction to the case

A patient had recently received a dual-chamber PM after mitral valve replacement. A peroperative fluoroscopic image is shown in Figure 13.1.

Question

Figure 13.1 Fluoroscopic image of the leads shown in 33° LAO projection

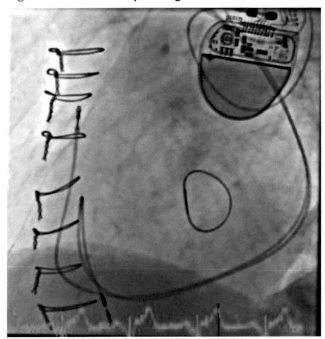

Which route of implant best describes the X-ray image?

A Inadvertent placement in the coronary sinus via the right atrium (RA)

B Inadvertent implantation via a patent foramen ovale

C Lead implantation via a persistent left superior vena cava (SVC)

D Normal transvenous route from left subclavian vein to the RA and right ventricle (RV)

E Through the right subclavian vein due to surgical closure of the left subclavian vein

Answer

C Lead implantation via a persistent left superior vena cava (SVC)

Figure 13.2 Annotated image

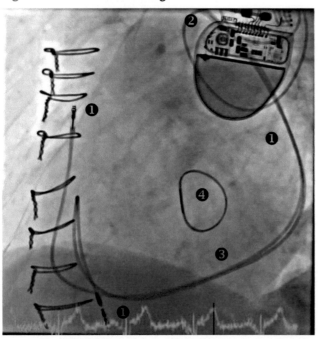

❶ Both leads are screw-in leads following the same transvenous route, and do not enter the cardiac chambers via a right-sided SVC (Figure 13.2).

❷ The take-off is relatively early, which is typical for a persistent left SVC. The generator is on the right of the image in the left anterior oblique (LAO) view, and is therefore placed in the left hemithorax.

❸ The leads follow the normal path for the coronary sinus in the LAO projection, and into the RA. The RV lead then passed through the tricuspid valve into the RV and the RA lead to the lateral wall of the RA.

❹ Annuloplasty ring in the mitral valve position.

Comments

Persistent left superior vena cava

The prevalence of persistent left superior vena cava (PLSVC) is estimated to be around 0.5%, and it is thus a condition that all device implanters must learn to recognize and handle accordingly. Often PLSVC is seen with absence of the left innominate vein, with either a double SVC with both PLSVC and right SVC or with complete atresia of the right SVC system.

Figure 13.3 Posteroanterior fluoroscopic images stored during device implantation. (a) Venogram showing the PLSVC and absence of a left innominate vein. (b) Final lead position

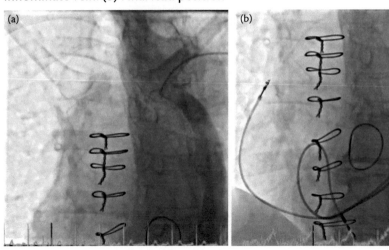

Implanting standard PM leads is most often feasible through the PLSVC, although directing the lead from the coronary sinus to the RV can be challenging. With the stiffer defibrillator lead, this may be even more difficult.

It is often not feasible to implant the RA lead in the RA appendage, and a position on the lateral wall may have to be accepted.

In case of CRT implantation, it is usually preferable to opt for a right-sided approach (if a right-sided SVC is present), as it can be very difficult to place and obtain a stable position in the target vessel via a PLSVC.

References

1. Chen X, Yu Z, Bai J, et al. Transvenous cardiac implantable electronic device implantation in patients with persistent left superior vena cava in a tertiary center. *J Interv Card Electrophysiol* 2018; **53**: 255–62.
2. Bontempi L, Aboelhassan M, Cerini M, et al. Technical considerations for CRT-D implantation in different varieties of persistent left superior vena cava. *J Interv Card Electrophysiol* 2021; **61**: 517–24.

Introduction to the case

A patient awaiting AVN ablation for rapidly conducted AF had a PM implanted. The real-time EGM during device interrogation on the day following implantation is shown in Figure 14.1.

Question

Figure 14.1 Real-time EGM recording at device follow-up on the day after PM implantation

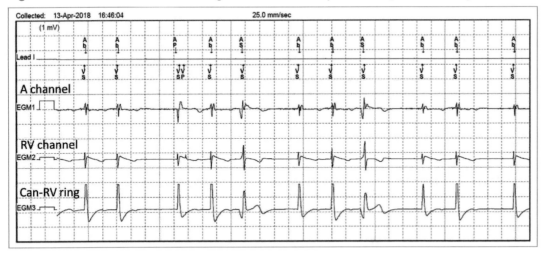

What is the most likely diagnosis?

A Atrial lead dislodged to the ventricle

B His lead connected to the atrial port

C Ventricular safety pacing

D A and C are correct

E B and C are correct

Answer

E B and C are correct

Figure 14.2 Annotated tracing

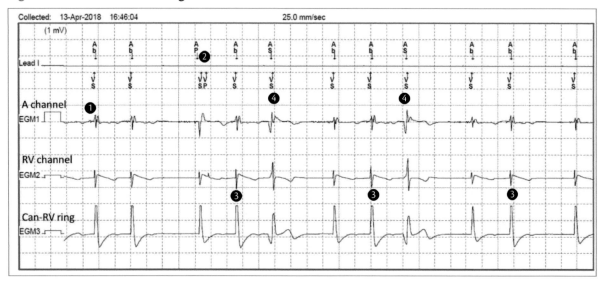

The patient had undergone implantation of a His lead connected to the atrial channel, with a backup RV lead and was awaiting AVN ablation for rapidly conducted AF.

❶ His potential visible on His lead connected to atrial port with simultaneous ventricular EGMs on the atrial and RV channels (Figure 14.2).

❷ Pacing from the atrial channel resulting in a QRS complex with identical morphology in the ventricular and far-field channels as compared to during VS (morphology would have been different in the case of atrial lead dislodgment to the ventricle). Ventricular safety pacing due to sensing in the ventricular channel occurring within 110 ms of pacing from the atrial channel.

❸ Slight aberrancy in intraventricular conduction due to long–short sequence (Ashman phenomenon).

❹ Ventricular premature beat with sensing on His lead before RV lead, change in near-field and far-field EGM morphology, no His potential preceding the event.

Comments

His bundle pacing lead connected to the atrial port

Current devices are not designed for His bundle pacing (HBP). HBP in patients in AF who have backup VP (or an additional implantable cardioverter defibrillator (ICD) lead), require the His lead to be connected to the atrial port. Backup VP is an option in patients undergoing AVN ablation for rapidly conducted AF, due to the risk of increased His capture thresholds resulting from the ablation.[1, 2] This will, however, result in unnecessary ventricular safety pacing as the delay between HBP and RV sensing is 85 ± 25 ms and falls within the ventricular safety pacing window (95–110 ms, depending upon the manufacturer).[3] Ventricular safety pacing can be inactivated in most devices, but this should be done after having ruled out crosstalk (i.e. sensing of the AP spike on the ventricular channel, with inhibition of VP, which may be lethal in case of complete AVB).[4]

References

1. Vijayaraman P, Subzposh FA, Naperkowski A. Atrioventricular node ablation and His bundle pacing. *Europace* 2017; **19**: iv10–16.
2. Zweerink A, Bakelants E, Stettler C, Burri H. Cryoablation vs. radiofrequency ablation of the atrioventricular node in patients with His-bundle pacing. *Europace* 2021; **23**: 421–30.
3. Starr N, Dayal N, Domenichini G, Stettler C, Burri H. Electrical parameters with His-bundle pacing: considerations for automated programming. *Heart Rhythm* 2019; **16**: 1817–24.
4. Burri H, Keene D, Whinnett Z, Zanon F, Vijayaraman P. Device programming for His bundle pacing. *Circ Arrhythm Electrophysiol* 2019; **12**: e006816.

Introduction to the case

A 12-lead ECG recorded during a threshold test in a patient implanted with HBP is shown in Figure 15.1.

Question

Figure 15.1 ECG recorded during the threshold test of the His lead

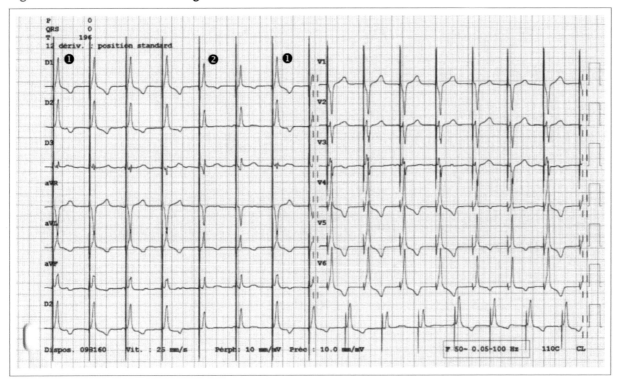

What can be observed?

A Intermittent loss of bundle branch correction

B Intermittent loss of His bundle capture

C Intermittent loss of myocardial capture

D The patient is PM dependent

E Variation in QRS amplitude due to respiration

Answer

C Intermittent loss of myocardial capture

Figure 15.2 Annotated tracing

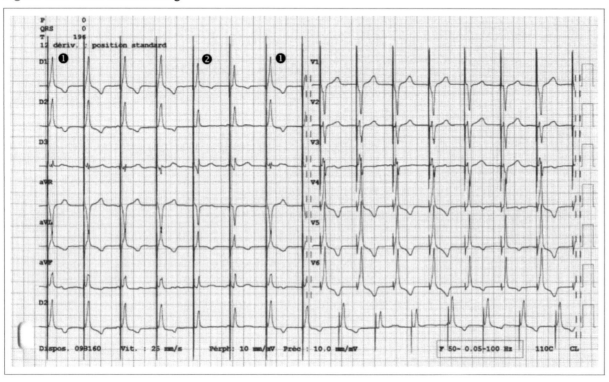

❶ The first four cycles and the last cycle are non-selective His bundle pacing (ns-HBP), that is, with both His and myocardial capture (Figure 15.2). Myocardial capture is visible as a 'pseudo-delta' wave mimicking a para-Hisian accessory pathway. Note that a pseudo-delta wave is not clearly visible in some leads (V2, V3) due to a perpendicular wavefront.

❷ This and the next cycle are selective His bundle pacing (s-HBP), that is, with loss of myocardial capture and His bundle capture only. Note the iso-electric interval in all 12 leads, corresponding to the HV interval. The fall in R-wave amplitude in leads I, II, and V6 is typical for transitions from ns-HBP to s-HBP (and may more clearly show the transition than disappearance of a small pseudo-delta wave).

Comments

His bundle pacing with selective and non-selective capture

Depending on the position of the lead and the presence of surrounding myocardium, HBP may capture myocardium as well as conduction tissue (Figure 15.3).[1] Capture of ventricular myocardium alters the initial portion of the QRS complex with a 'pseudo-delta' wave.

Figure 15.3 Schematic representation of His bundle lead insertion and s-HBP and ns-HBP. In case of proximal insertion without surrounding myocardial sleeves, pacing is obligatory s-HBP. The amplitude and duration of the pseudo-delta wave will depend upon the mass of surrounding myocardium being captured as well as the HV interval (larger pseudo-delta wave in case of prolonged HV)

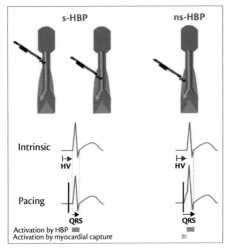

Reproduced from Burri H, Jastrzębski M, Vijayaraman P. Electrocardiographic Analysis for His Bundle Pacing at Implantation and Follow-Up. *JACC Clin Electrophysiol.* 2020 Jul;6(7):883–900. doi: 10.1016/j.jacep.2020.03.005 with permission from Elsevier.

ns-HBP offers the advantage of backup myocardial capture in case of loss of His capture but may result in less synchronous ventricular activation than s-HBP.

Reference

1. Burri H, Jastrzębski M, Vijayaraman P. Electrocardiographic analysis for His bundle pacing at implantation and follow-up. *JACC Clin Electrophysiol* 2020; **6**: 883–900.

Introduction to the case

A capture threshold test was performed in a patient in chronic AF awaiting AVN ablation. A His lead had been implanted and was connected to the atrial port, with a backup RV lead connected to the ventricular port. The real-time EGM during the threshold test is shown in Figure 16.1.

Question

Figure 16.1 Real-time EGM during the capture threshold test of the His lead (connected to the atrial port of the PM)

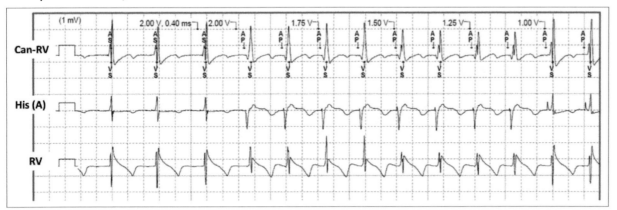

Which of the following is true?

A His capture threshold is 1.25 V/0.4 ms

B Myocardial capture threshold is 1.25 V

C Patient has obligatory selective capture

D Transition is from non-selective to myocardial capture

E Transition is from selective to non-selective His capture

Answer

B Myocardial capture threshold is 1.25 V

Figure 16.2 Annotated tracing (His lead connected to the atrial port and RV channels are in the bipolar configuration)

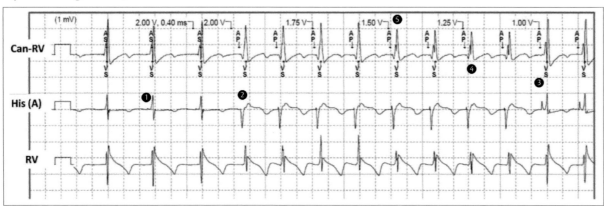

❶ The first three cycles are in intrinsic rhythm, with sensing in the atrial channel (His lead) occurring just before the ventricular channel (Figure 16.2). A tiny His potential is visible in the second and third cycles.

❷ The threshold test is initiated, with decrementing output and initial ns-HBP. The His lead EGM shows a prominently negative morphology, with changes in EGM morphology in the far-field (can-RV) and RV channels compared to intrinsic rhythm.

❸ Loss of myocardial capture, with s-HBP for the last two cycles of the tracing (loss of local myocardial capture). Note the iso-electric interval between the pacing spike and ventricular deflection, corresponding to the HV interval. The far-field and RV EGM morphologies are identical to those in intrinsic rhythm.

❹ Transient ventricular undersensing (for two cycles). The sensitivity of the ventricular channel needs to be increased.

❺ Slight change in EGM morphology, possible due to loss of correction of bundle branch block at 1.5 V.

Comments

Electrogram analysis of non-selective and selective His bundle pacing

A negative deflection after pacing on the His lead indicates ns-HBP or myocardial capture, as does a time to peak deflection of <40 ms, with sensitivity and specificity of ≥90%.[1] Changes in EGM morphology as shown in this example are very useful for detecting transitions from ns-HBP to s-HBP (as the pseudo-delta wave may not always be apparent, or if a 12-lead ECG is not available).

When the His lead is connected to the LV channel of Medtronic CRT devices, the EffectivCRT algorithm (designed to distinguish identify beats with LV non-capture) labels cycles with a QS complex (ns-HBP or myocardial capture) as being 'effective' capture, and other cycles as being 'ineffective' capture (including cycles with s-HBP, see Figure 16.3).

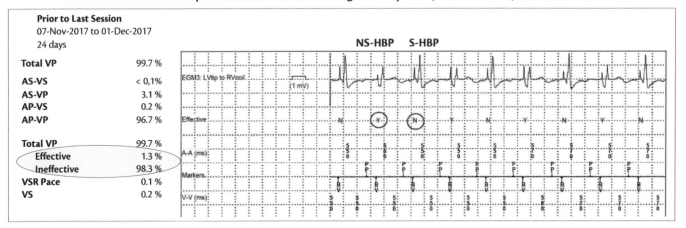

Figure 16.3 EffectivCRT algorithm in patients with a His lead connected to the LV port, which identifies complexes with ns-HBP and a 'QS' complex as being capture (labelled as 'Y'), and s-HBP with an isoelectric interval and a positive deflection, as being non-capture (labelled as 'N')

Reference

1. Saini A, Serafini NJ, Campbell S, et al. Novel method for assessment of His bundle pacing morphology using near field and far field device electrograms. *Circ Arrhythm Electrophysiol* 2019; **12**: e006878.

Introduction to the case

A 12-lead ECG was recorded in a patient with HBP during a capture threshold test and is shown in Figure 17.1.

Question

Figure 17.1 ECG recorded in a patient with HBP during a threshold test

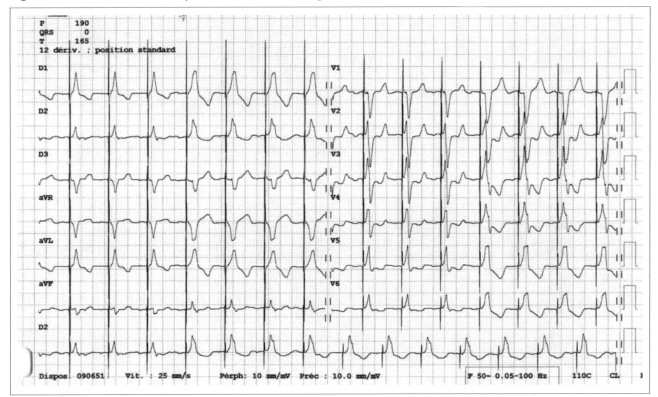

The transition in QRS morphology is due to:

A Loss of atrial capture

B Loss of bundle branch correction

C Loss of His capture

D Loss of myocardial capture

E Rate-related aberrancy

Answer

C Loss of His capture

Figure 17.2 Annotated tracing

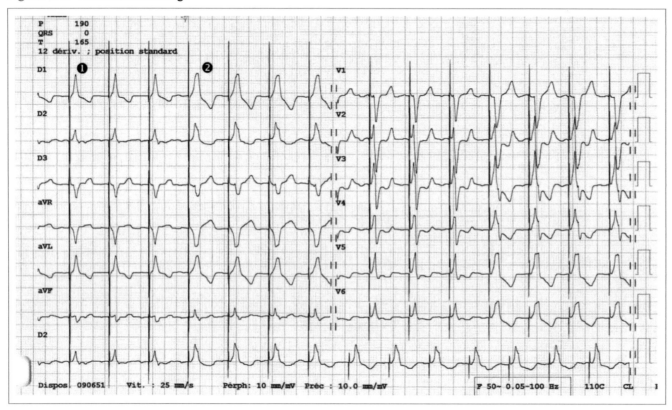

In Figure 17.2, a sudden broadening of the QRS complex is visible with decrementing output, corresponding to transition from ns-HBP to myocardial capture only.

❶ The first three QRS complexes correspond to ns-HBP.

❷ From this point on, capture is myocardial only (loss of His capture).

Comments

His and myocardial thresholds and QRS transitions

Depending on the respective thresholds of His and surrounding myocardium, transitions vary (Figure 17.3).

Figure 17.3 Transitions with decrementing pacing output in patients with a normal baseline QRS. (a) Obligatory s-HBP in patients without surrounding myocardium (no transition). (b) Transition from ns-HBP → s-HBP (loss of myocardial capture). (c) Transition from ns-HBP → myocardial capture (loss of His capture)

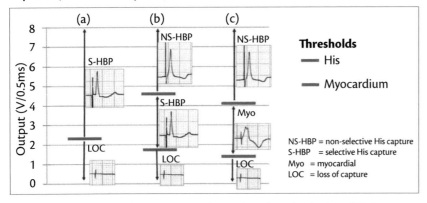

Reproduced from Burri H, Jastrzębski M, Vijayaraman P. Electrocardiographic Analysis for His Bundle Pacing at Implantation and Follow-Up. *JACC Clin Electrophysiol.* 2020 Jul;6(7):883–900. doi: 10.1016/j.jacep.2020.03.005 with permission from Elsevier.

This example also serves to show the features which distinguish ns-HBP from myocardial capture only (Figure 17.4).[1,2]

Figure 17.4 Morphological features to distinguish ns-HBP from myocardial capture (Myo). Notches, slurring, and plateaus may nevertheless be observed with ns-HBP in patients with underlying left bundle branch block or non-specific interventricular conduction delay (RWPT, R-wave peak time)

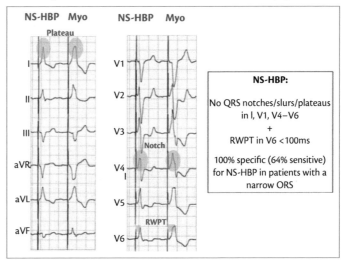

Reproduced from Burri H, Jastrzębski M, Vijayaraman P. Electrocardiographic Analysis for His Bundle Pacing at Implantation and Follow-Up. *JACC Clin Electrophysiol.* 2020 Jul;6(7):883–900. doi: 10.1016/j.jacep.2020.03.005 with permission from Elsevier.

References

1. Jastrzebski M, Moskal P, Curila K, et al. Electrocardiographic characterization of non-selective His-bundle pacing: validation of novel diagnostic criteria. *Europace* 2019; **21**: 1857–64.
2. Burri H, Jastrzębski M, Vijayaraman P. Electrocardiographic analysis for His bundle pacing at implantation and follow-up. *JACC Clin Electrophysiol* 2020; **6**: 883–900.

Introduction to the case

An ECG was recorded during implantation of a His lead while pacing at 2.5 V/1 ms unipolar in a patient with left bundle branch block (LBBB) at baseline (Figure 18.1).

Question

Figure 18.1 ECG recorded at His lead implantation while pacing at 2.5 V/1 ms (unipolar), showing four morphologies of captured beats

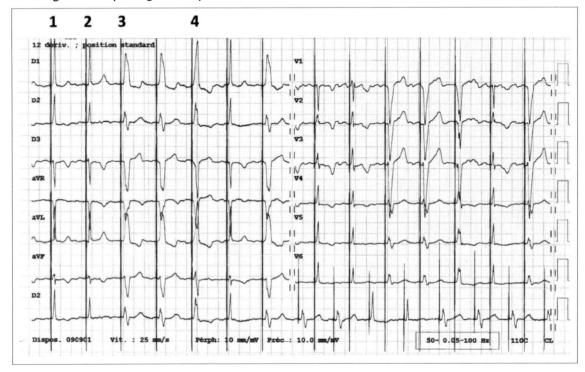

Which beat corresponds to ns-HBP with correction of LBBB?

A 1

B 2

C 3

D 4

E LBBB is not corrected

Answer

A 1

Figure 18.2 Annotated tracing

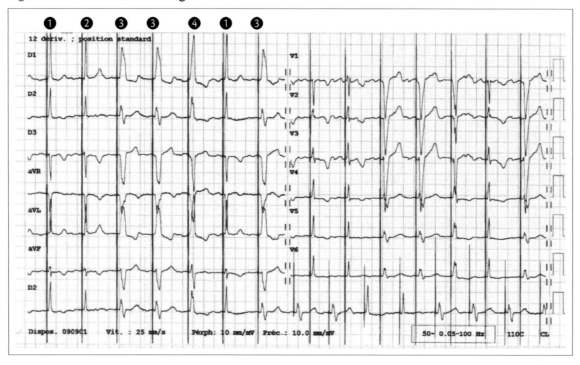

❶ ns-HBP with correction of LBBB is present in the first and sixth beats (Figure 18.2). Note the narrow QRS with a pseudo-delta wave in lead I.

❷ s-HBP with correction of LBBB. The QRS is narrow, with an iso-electric interval between the pacing spike and QRS onset. Note the reduction in R-wave amplitude in leads I, II, and V6 compare to the preceding cycle, typical of a transition from ns-HBP to s-HBP.

❸ s-HBP without correction of LBBB is present in the third, fourth, and last beats. Note the iso-electric interval in all 12 leads and typical LBBB pattern, which was identical to the intrinsic rhythm.

❹ Myocardial capture only or ns-HBP without correction of LBBB.

Comments

His bundle pacing in patients with bundle branch block

It has been shown since the late 1970s that HBP can correct LBBB and right bundle branch block (RBBB) in a subset of patients, implying longitudinal dissociation of conduction within the His bundle,[1,2] and intra-Hisian site of block (46% of patients with LBBB[3]). If the His lead is placed distally to the site of block, the BBB may be corrected (Figure 18.3).

Figure 18.3 Presence or absence of correction of bundle branch block (BBB) depending upon the level of block and implantation site of the His lead

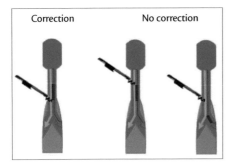

In this patient, thresholds for the myocardium, His bundle, and correction of LBBB were very close, leading to different QRS morphologies over consecutive cycles at the same pacing output (probably due to slight differences in lead orientation). At implantation, thresholds may be dynamic due to regression of current of injury and different transitions may be observed during the course of the procedure (Figure 18.4).

Figure 18.4 Types of transitions with decrementing pacing output, depending upon respective thresholds of correction of BBB, His bundle capture, and myocardial capture

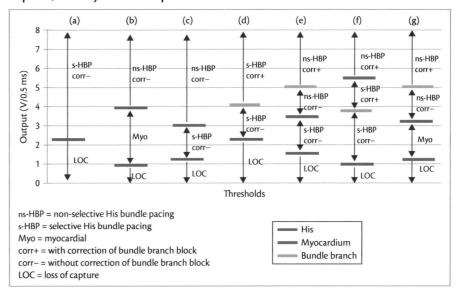

ns-HBP = non-selective His bundle pacing
s-HBP = selective His bundle pacing
Myo = myocardial
corr+ = with correction of bundle branch block
corr− = without correction of bundle branch block
LOC = loss of capture

— His
— Myocardium
— Bundle branch

References

1. Narula OS. Longitudinal dissociation in the His bundle. Bundle branch block due to asynchronous conduction within the His bundle in man. *Circulation* 1977; **56**: 996–1006.
2. El-Sherif N, Amay YLF, Schonfield C, et al. Normalization of bundle branch block patterns by distal His bundle pacing. Clinical and experimental evidence of longitudinal dissociation in the pathologic his bundle. *Circulation* 1978; **57**: 473–83.
3. Upadhyay GA, Cherian T, Shatz DY, et al. Intracardiac delineation of septal conduction in left bundle-branch block patterns. *Circulation* 2019; **139**: 1876–88.

Introduction to the case

A 12-lead ECG was recorded in a patient with HBP during a capture threshold test at implantation and is shown in Figure 19.1. The patient had underlying RBBB.

Question

Figure 19.1 ECG recorded in a patient with HBP during a threshold test

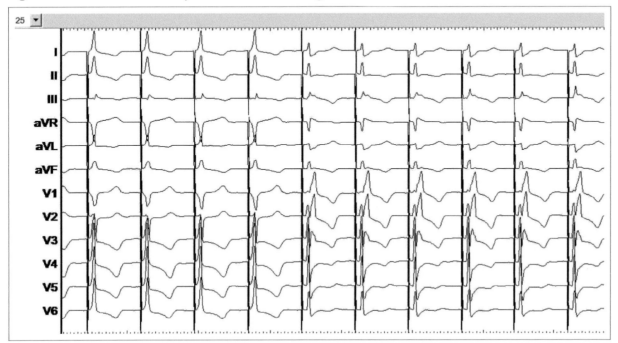

The transition in QRS morphology is most likely due to:

A Loss of atrial capture

B Loss of bundle branch correction

C Loss of His capture

D Loss of myocardial capture

E None of the above

Answer

D Loss of myocardial capture

Figure 19.2 Annotated tracing

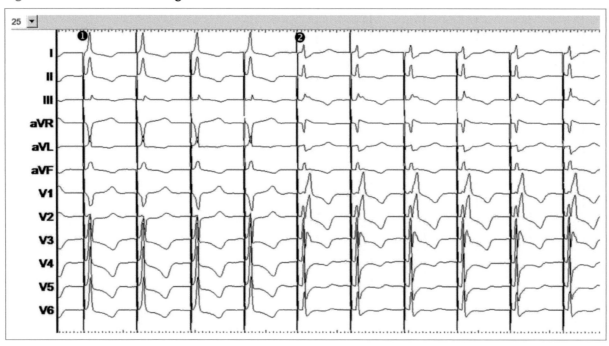

A sudden broadening of the QRS complex is visible in Figure 19.2 with decrementing output, corresponding to transition from ns-HBP to s-HBP with uncorrected RBBB.

❶ The first four QRS complexes correspond to ns-HBP. A pseudo-delta wave is clearly visible (e.g. in leads I, V3–V6). Correction of RBBB cannot be excluded, but it is unlikely to be lost at the same time as myocardial capture.

❷ From this point on, capture is s-HBP with uncorrected RBBB (loss of myocardial capture). Note the iso-electric interval in all 12 leads.

Comments

Effect of myocardial capture in non-selective His bundle pacing in patients with underlying bundle branch block

This patient has a transition corresponding to (c) in Figure 18.4 in Case 18.

Much as fusion of intrinsic conduction with LV pacing narrows the QRS in CRT patients with LBBB, fusion of His activation and RV myocardial capture in patients with underlying RBBB also serves to narrow the QRS (Figure 19.3). Conversely, in patients with uncorrected LBBB, ns-HBP can widen the QRS complex.

Figure 19.3 Effect on QRS duration by ns-HBP without correction of BBB (lead I is depicted here). The QRS is shortened in the setting of RBBB and lengthened with LBBB

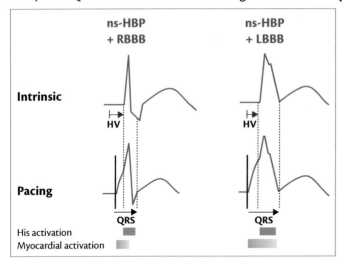

It is difficult to diagnose correction of RBBB in the setting of ns-HBP. Presence of terminal conduction abnormalities such as an S-wave in lead I and an Qr pattern in V1 may indicate underlying uncorrected RBBB.[1]

Reference

1. Burri H, Jastrzębski M, Vijayaraman P. Electrocardiographic analysis for His bundle pacing at implantation and follow-up. *JACC Clin Electrophysiol* 2020; **6**: 883–900.

Introduction to the case

A patient with paroxysmal AVB was implanted with a PM with HBP. An ECG recorded during a threshold test on the day following implantation is shown in Figure 20.1.

Question

Figure 20.1 ECG recording during a threshold test from the His lead

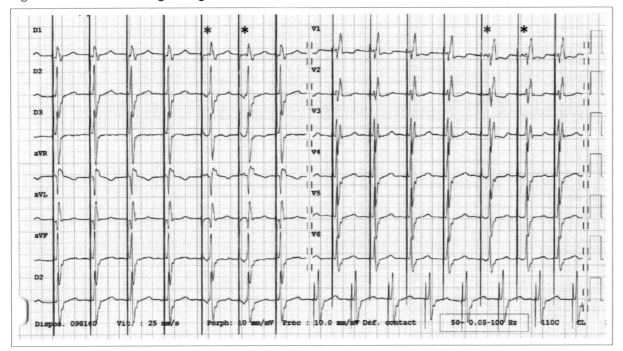

How do you explain the prolongation of the stimulus–QRS interval in two cycles shown by the asterisks?

A Backup VP

B HV prolongation

C Loss of bundle branch correction

D Loss of His capture

E Loss of myocardial capture

Answer

D Loss of His capture

Figure 20.2 Annotated tracing

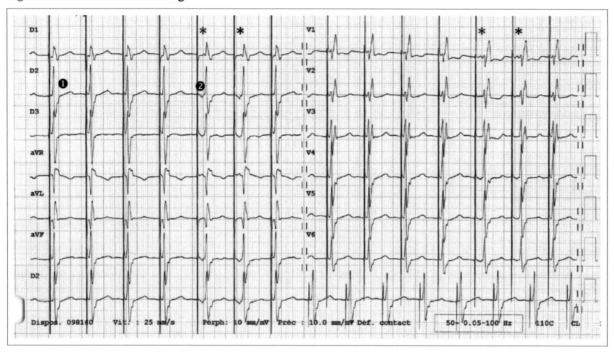

The tracing was recorded while pacing at an output close to the His threshold with intermittent loss of His capture for the two beats indicated by the asterisks (capture resumes for the last beat) (Figure 20.2).

❶ The first four and last beats show s-HBP without correction of RBBB. Atrial capture is also present, but is invisible.

❷ Loss of His capture, with persistence of atrial capture and AV conduction, resulting in a prolongation of stimulus–QRS interval. The morphology of the QRS complex remains unchanged.

Comments

Atrial capture with His bundle pacing

When the His lead is implanted relatively proximally, atrial capture can be observed (Figure 20.3).

Figure 20.3 Transient loss of His/myocardial capture (fourth spike), with persistence of atrial capture (and AVB)

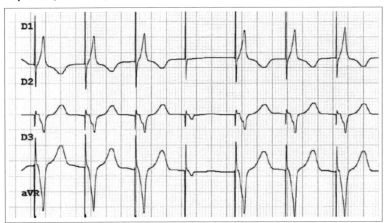

Atrial capture may confound capture threshold measurements in case of preserved AV conduction if the stimulus–QRS delay prolongation is not identified (Figure 20.4).

Figure 20.4 Threshold test with atrial capture, which should not be mistaken for s-HBP, with erroneous threshold values. Note that in this example, both atrial and ventricular myocardium are captured

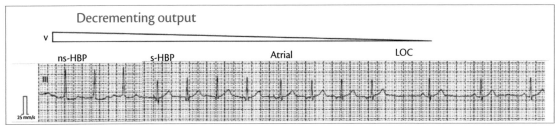

Also, loss of atrial capture may masquerade as transitions in QRS morphology (Figure 20.5).

Figure 20.5 At high output from the His lead (left), there is ns-HBP with atrial capture (no visible P-wave due to simultaneous capture). With lower output (right), atrial capture is lost, with retrograde conduction masquerading as an S-wave in the inferior leads (shaded circles)

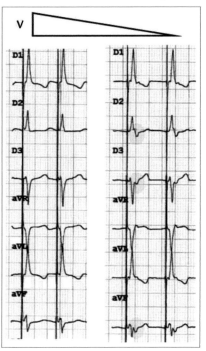

Introduction to the case

A patient in chronic AF with AVN ablation and HBP had programmed stimulation from the His bundle lead (Figure 21.1).

Question

Figure 21.1 Programmed pacing from the His lead at a drive cycle of 600 ms and paced premature beat of 310 ms

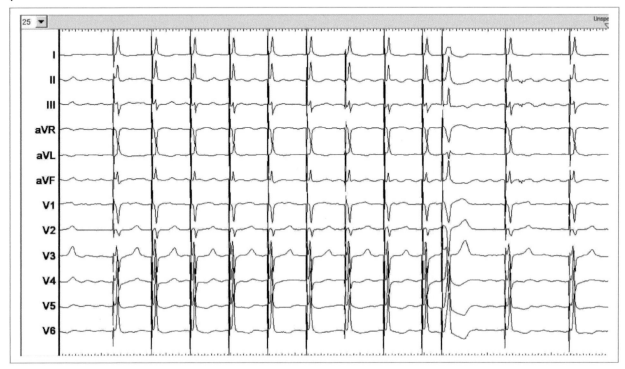

What do you observe with the paced premature beat?

A Latency

B Loss of His capture

C Loss of myocardial capture

D Pacing from a backup LV lead

E Pacing from a backup RV lead

Answer

B Loss of His capture

Figure 21.2 Annotated tracing

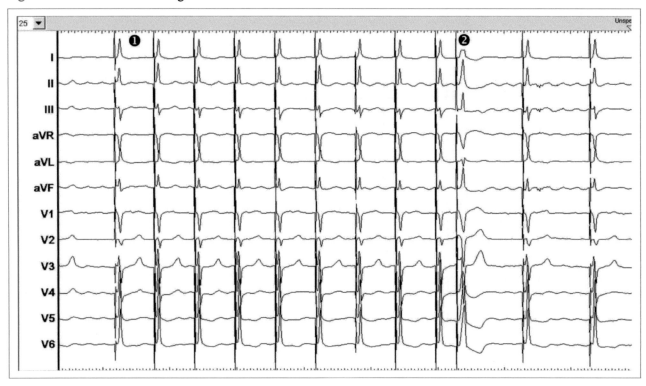

❶ The beats of the drive cycle at 600 ms (100 bpm) and the last two cycles show ns-HBP (note the pseudo-delta wave) (Figure 21.2). Latency refers to an iso-electrical line in all 12 leads between the pacing spike and QRS onset, which is absent in this example.

❷ The premature beat at 310 ms (193 bpm) falls in the refractory period of the His bundle, with myocardial capture only.

Comments

Programmed His pacing

This technique can be used to distinguish ns-HBP from myocardial capture only, which is particularly useful when the His and myocardial thresholds are almost identical and cannot be distinguished by decrementing pacing output. The technique exploits differences in refractory periods between the His bundle and myocardial tissue (the former being longer in 94% of patients, with average refractory periods of the His bundle being 353 ± 30 ms and that of the myocardium being 272 ± 38 ms at drive cycles of 600 ms[1]). Alternatives to programmed pacing with extra beats is burst pacing (Figure 21.3) and pacing in the VOO mode to sample different coupling intervals.

Figure 21.3 Burst pacing from the His lead at a cycle length of 390 ms. The QRS complexes which are covered by the arrow are wide due to myocardial capture only. The refractory period of the His bundle shortens over consecutive beats, with resumption of ns-HBP thereafter

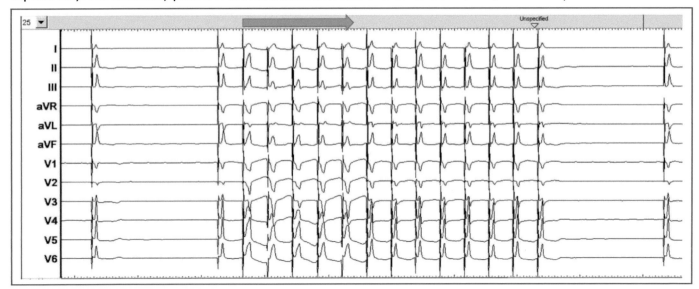

Caveats of programmed stimulation are widening of the QRS complex due to aberrant conduction and decremental His–Purkinje conduction (which masquerade as myocardial capture). Furthermore, in case of myocardial capture only during the drive cycles, the extrasystolic beat may show slight changes in QRS morphology due to intramyocardial delay and should not be interpreted as a transition due to loss of His capture.[2]

References

1. Jastrzębski M, Moskal P, Bednarek A, Kielbasa G, Vijayaraman P, Czarnecka D. Programmed His bundle pacing. *Circ Arrhythm Electrophysiol* 2019; **12**: e007052.
2. Burri H, Jastrzębski M, Vijayaraman P. Electrocardiographic analysis for His bundle pacing at implantation and follow-up. *JACC Clin Electrophysiol* 2020; **6**: 883–900.

Introduction to the case

A capture threshold test was performed in a patient with AVB and a DDD PM with an atrial lead and a His lead connected to the ventricular port. The real-time tracing during decrementing output from the His lead is shown in Figure 22.1.

Question

Figure 22.1 Real-time EGM during the capture threshold test of the His lead (connected to the ventricular port of the PM)

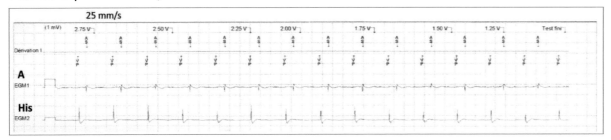

What is the His capture threshold?

A 2.25 V

B 2.0 V

C 1.75 V

D 1.5 V

E 1.25 V

Answer

C 1.75 V

Figure 22.2 Annotated tracing

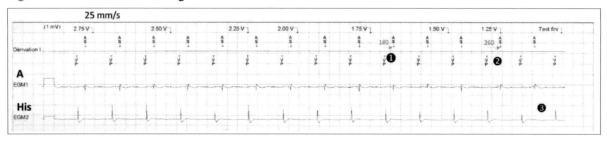

❶ 1:1 retrograde conduction is seen from the onset of His pacing with a stimulus–A interval which remains constant at 180 ms down to 1.75 V (Figure 22.2).

❷ At 1.5 V, the stimulus–A interval suddenly prolongs at the second cycle to 260 ms and remains constant thereafter. This corresponds to loss of His capture (transition from ns-HBP to myocardial capture only). As the capture threshold refers to output resulting in consistent capture, the His threshold is therefore 1.75 V.

❸ The His EGM morphology remains constant throughout the tracing as there is local myocardial capture (with an initial negative deflection), except for the very last cycle (which probably corresponds to loss of myocardial capture).

Comments

Electrogram analysis of stimulus–A intervals to diagnose loss of His capture

In patients who have preserved VA conduction, a sudden increase in stimulus–A interval implies loss of His capture (Figure 22.3).

Figure 22.3 Prolongation of stimulus–A interval with loss of His capture (transition from ns-HBP to myocardial capture) in patients with preserved VA conduction

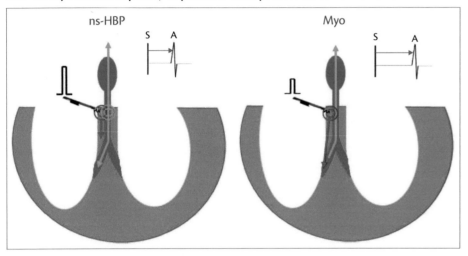

This observation is similar to para-Hisian pacing performed in the electrophysiology laboratory to evaluate the presence of a septal accessory pathway. A caveat is atrial capture by the His lead at high pacing output which shortens the stimulus–A interval, with sudden lengthening of the interval when atrial capture is lost by decrementing the output.

Introduction to the case

A patient with complete AVB had been recently implanted with a dual-chamber PM with an atrial lead and a His lead. He presented with bouts of lightheadedness. A real-time EGM during in-office follow-up is shown in Figure 23.1. The patient was asymptomatic at that moment. The programmed parameters are shown in Table 23.1.

Table 23.1 Programmed parameters

Mode	DDD 50–130 bpm
AV delay (sensed/paced)	120/150 ms
Atrial channel:	
Sensing	0.3 mV (bipolar)
Pacing	2.5 V/0.4 ms (bipolar)
Ventricular (His) channel:	
Sensing	0.9 mV (bipolar)
Pacing	2.5 V/0.4 ms (bipolar)
PVARP	Auto
PVAB	150 ms
PAVB	30 ms

Question

Figure 23.1 Real-time EGM during follow-up

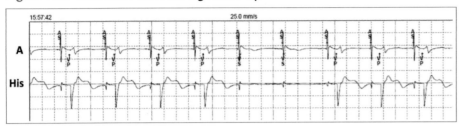

What do you observe?

A Atrial double counting

B FFRW oversensing

C His non-capture

D Oversensing by the His lead (ventricular channel)

E Ventricular safety pacing is inactivated

Answer

D Oversensing by the His lead (ventricular channel)

Figure 23.2 Annotated tracing

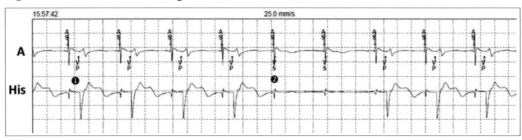

The tracing in Figure 23.2 shows transient non-pacing from the His lead (ventricular channel) with a pause of approximately 2 s, due to sensing of atrial potentials.

❶ The first four and last three beats show AS followed by HBP with non-selective His (or myocardial) capture, as indicated by QS morphology of the captured EGM. A small FFRW is visible on the atrial channel but is not sensed (no marker is displayed). A small atrial potential is also visible on the His lead but is not sensed in these cycles.

❷ The atrial potential on the His lead is sensed for two cycles (VS markers), leading to inhibition of pacing.

It is impossible to determine whether ventricular safety pacing is activated or not, as it is triggered by AP only (and not sensing).

Comments

Sensing issues with His bundle pacing

Sensing issues are encountered more frequently with His leads than with standard ventricular leads, especially when the lead is implanted in a proximal position (on the atrial aspect of the tricuspid valve). Ventricular undersensing can occur due to the 'far-field' ventricular signal. Atrial and His potential oversensing can also occur and may be disastrous in a PM-dependent patient.[1] Troubleshooting of the atrial oversensing issue in this case is shown in Figures 23.3 and 23.4.

Figure 23.3 Sensing test of the ventricular (His) channel with the sensitivity set to 0.6 mV (bipolar) and temporary VVI 30 bpm pacing showing complete AVB and a ventricular escape rhythm with consistent oversensing of atrial potentials on the His lead. VS amplitude was measured automatically at 0.8 mV. Note, however, that this amplitude corresponds to the atrial potential, and that the ventricular potential is much larger according to the scale marker (the device yielded the value of the lowest measured amplitude)

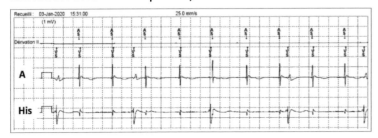

Figure 23.4 The sensing test is repeated with ventricular (His) channel sensitivity set at 1.2 mV (bipolar), without atrial oversensing, and with measured ventricular amplitude of 2.1 mV

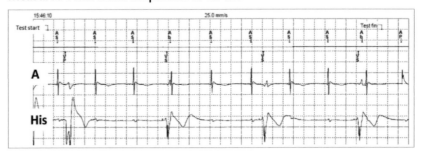

The device was finally programmed with bipolar sensitivity of 1.2 mV.

Unipolar sensing could also have been tested to evaluate P-wave oversensing, but carries a risk of pectoral muscle oversensing in this PM-dependent patient.

Adjusting post-atrial ventricular blanking (PAVB) is not helpful as this only applies to AP events. Backup ventricular leads sometimes need to be implanted for adequate ventricular sensing in the setting of HBP.

Reference

1. Burri H, Keene D, Whinnett Z, Zanon F, Vijayaraman P. Device programming for His bundle pacing. *Circ Arrhythm Electrophysiol* 2019; **12**: e006816.

Introduction to the case

A patient with infranodal 2:1 AVB (Figure 24.1) was implanted with a dual-chamber PM with an atrial lead and a left bundle branch area pacing (LBBAP) lead. Her ECG during a threshold test performed during implantation in a unipolar pacing configuration is shown in Figure 24.2.

Figure 24.1 Mapping of the His bundle with the pacing lead prior to LBBAP implantation showing 2:1 infranodal block (HIS F, filtered His; HIS NF, non-filtered HIS)

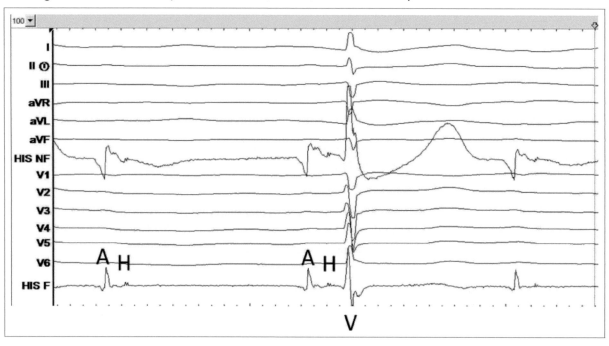

Question

Figure 24.2   Threshold test at implantation of the LBBAP lead with decrementing output in the unipolar configuration (loss of capture occurred at 0.7 V/0.5 ms)

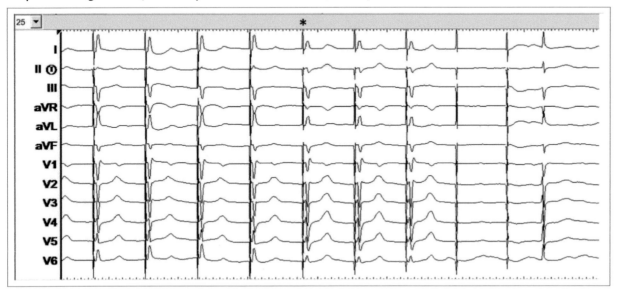

What event is denoted by the asterisk?

A Loss of anodal capture

B Loss of anterior fascicular capture

C Loss of left bundle branch (LBB) capture

D Loss of myocardial capture

E Loss of posterior fascicular capture

Answer

D Loss of myocardial capture

Figure 24.3 Annotated tracing

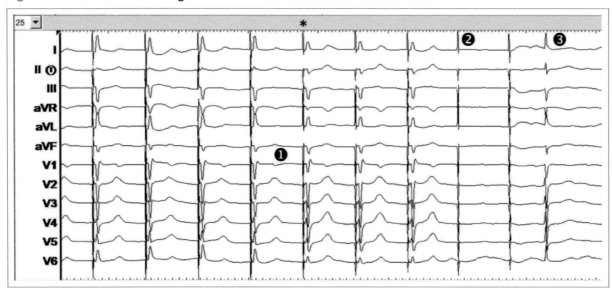

Anodal capture is impossible due to the unipolar pacing configuration.

❶ With loss of septal myocardial capture which fuses with LBB activation, the QRS complex assumes a RBBB morphology due to selective capture of the LBB (the left axis deviation implies that the lead was positioned on the posterior fascicle) (Figure 24.3). Note also the reduction in QRS amplitude in leads I and V6 with transition from non-selective to selective LBB capture (this finding is also observed with HBP). Contrary to HBP, the isoelectric interval with selective capture is barely noticeable due to the very short delay between the LBB potential and QRS onset (only about 10–20 ms, compared to approximately 40–60 ms with the HV interval).

❷ Loss of LBB capture occurs shortly after loss of myocardial capture, indicating that the respective thresholds are very close.

❸ Intrinsic rhythm (with 2:1 AV conduction).

Comments

Confirming left bundle branch capture

Contrary to what is observed with HBP, transitions in QRS morphology with decrementing pacing output is observed in <20% of cases of LBBAP and is seldom useful for confirming LBB capture.[1]

This may be for a number of reasons:

1 Capture thresholds of the myocardium and LBB may be very close (as in the present case).
2 There is myocardial capture only (without conduction system capture).
3 There is retrograde activation of Purkinje tissue adjacent to the captured myocardium (i.e. secondary activation of the conduction system which depends upon myocardial capture).

Pacing manoeuvres similar to those used for HBP[2] which exploit differences in refractory periods between conduction tissue and the ventricular myocardium (cf. Case 21) may also be applied for confirming LBB capture.[1]

References

1. Jastrzębski M, Moskal P, Bednarek A, et al. Programmed deep septal stimulation: a novel maneuver for the diagnosis of left bundle branch capture during permanent pacing. *J Cardiovasc Electrophysiol* 2020; **31**: 485–93.
2. Jastrzębski M, Moskal P, Bednarek A, Kielbasa G, Vijayaraman P, Czarnecka D. Programmed his bundle pacing. *Circ Arrhythm Electrophysiol* 2019; **12**: e007052.

Introduction to the case

A patient with slowly conducted AF and LBBB was implanted with LBBAP. The ECG in intrinsic rhythm and with unipolar pacing is shown in Figure 25.1. A threshold test performed in the bipolar configuration is shown in Figure 25.2.

Figure 25.1 Intrinsic rhythm (left panel) and LBBAP at 10 V/0.5 ms in the unipolar configuration (right panel)

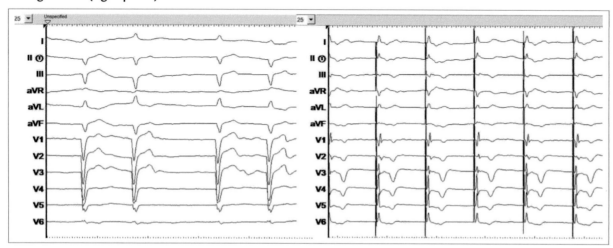

Question

Figure 25.2 Threshold test with bipolar pacing at 0.5 ms

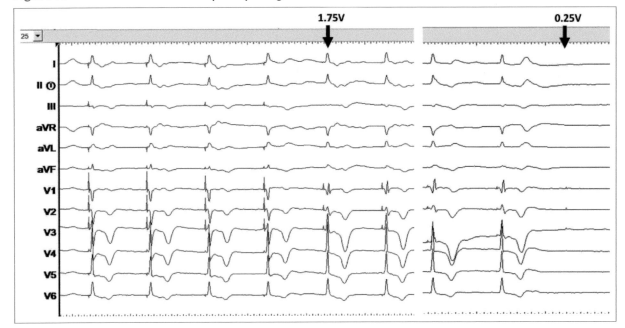

How do you explain the transition in QRS morphology at 1.75 V/0.5 ms?

A Loss of anodal capture

B Loss of anterior fascicular capture

C Loss of LBB capture

D Loss of myocardial capture

E Loss of posterior fascicular capture

Answer

A Loss of anodal capture

Figure 25.3 Annotated tracing

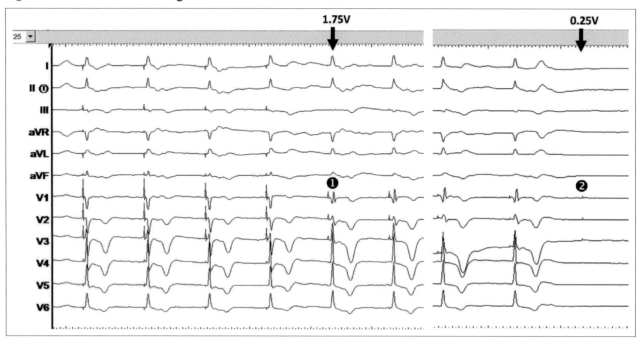

❶ The transition in QRS morphology corresponds to loss of anodal myocardial capture by the ring electrode embedded in the interventricular septum (Figure 25.3). The QRS morphology after loss of anodal capture is identical to that observed during unipolar pacing at 10 V/0.5 ms.

❷ Complete LOC occurs without any further transition in QRS morphology. This implies that the LBB and myocardial thresholds are almost identical, or that there is myocardial capture only. Selective capture of the LBB is unlikely due to the identical QRS morphology at 10 V/0.5 ms with unipolar pacing, which would be expected to result in myocardial capture.

Note the T-wave inversions due to cardiac memory of the pre-existent LBBB.

Comments

Anodal capture with left bundle branch area pacing

The ring electrode of the LBBAP lead is usually intramyocardial and can result in anodal capture when pacing in the bipolar mode. A transition in QRS morphology with loss of anodal capture can masquerade as a transition from non-selective to selective capture of the LBB. Anodal capture can be identified by comparing QRS morphologies during unipolar pacing at high output. Changes in EGM morphology are usually visible with loss of anodal capture (Figure 25.4).

Figure 25.4 Bipolar capture threshold test of the LBBAP lead in VVI mode in a patient with a dual-chamber pacemaker implanted for complete AVB. Change in RV tip-ring (EGM2) and generator-ring (EGM3) morphology with loss of anodal capture are visible at 1.75 V/0.4 ms (*). No further changes in morphology are visible until loss of capture at 0.25 V/0.4 ms. EGM1, right atrial channel

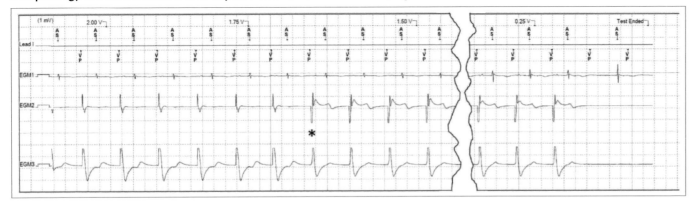

Impact on QRS morphology due to anodal capture can be observed in the following situations:

1. Pacing from a coronary sinus lead programmed in extended bipolar pacing configuration (LV tip to RV ring, or, more rarely, to RV coil—cf. Volume 1, Case 68)—resulting in simultaneous biventricular capture.
2. Biventricular pacing with the coronary sinus lead programmed in extended bipolar configuration, resulting in capture from the LV lead, and bifocal RV capture (triple site capture).[1]
3. Pacing from a coronary sinus lead programmed in a true bipolar pacing configuration with wide interelectrode spacing (thereby resulting in multipoint pacing).[2]
4. Pacing from a His bundle lead connected to the LV port of a CRT generator, programmed in extended bipolar pacing configuration with an RV backup lead.[3]
5. LBBAP programmed to bipolar pacing configuration (as in the present case).

References

1. Tamborero D, Mont L, Alanis R, et al. Anodal capture in cardiac resynchronization therapy implications for device programming. *Pacing Clin Electrophysiol* 2006; **29**: 940–5.
2. Occhetta E, Dell'Era G, Giubertoni A, et al. Occurrence of simultaneous cathodal-anodal capture with left ventricular quadripolar leads for cardiac resynchronization therapy: an electrocardiogram evaluation. *Europace* 2017; **19**: 596–601.
3. Starr N, Dayal N, Domenichini G, Stettler C, Burri H. Electrical parameters with His-bundle pacing: considerations for automated programming. *Heart Rhythm* 2019; **16**: 1817–24.

Introduction to the case

An 80-year-old patient received a leadless VVI PM for chronic AF with slow ventricular rate and intermittent dizziness. This device was preferred to a standard PM due to mechanical issues at both shoulders. A chest X-ray of the patient is shown in Figure 26.1.

Five years after implantation, the following measurements were obtained:

Electrode impedance: 630 Ohm.

Capture threshold: 2.13 V/0.24 ms.

Counters: VS 0.2%, VP 99.8%.

Battery voltage (RRT = 2.56 V): 2.59 V.

Parameter summary:

Mode: VVIR.

Lower rate: 60 bpm.

Upper sensor: 120 bpm.

Programmed amplitude/pulse width: 2.88 V /0.24 ms.

Question

Figure 26.1 Chest X-ray of a patient with a VVI PM system

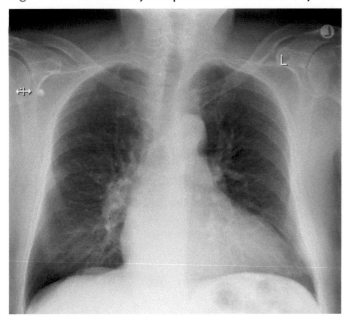

What is the most appropriate action when battery voltage reaches 2.56 V?

A Abandon the device and implant a new leadless pacemaker

B Abandon the device and implant a transvenous system

C Extract the device and implant a new leadless pacemaker

D Extract the device and implant a transvenous system

E Intensify follow-up visits to carefully monitor the battery voltage

Answer

A Abandon the device and implant a new leadless pacemaker

The device is a Medtronic Micra VR leadless device implanted in the apical region. The threshold was relatively high at implantation, causing a higher-than-expected battery drain for this device.

A new leadless device was easily implanted in the anteroseptal region with a low threshold (0.38 V/0.24 ms)—see Figure 26.2.

Figure 26.2 Annotated fluoroscopy during implantation of the new leadless PM (right anterior oblique projection)

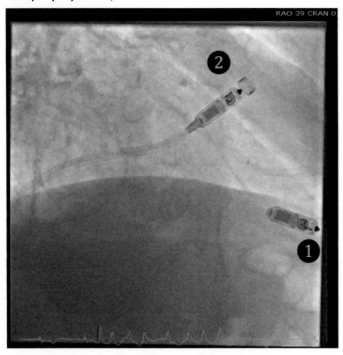

❶ First Micra VR leadless PM implanted in the apical region.

❷ New Micra leadless PM with delivery tool during implantation in the anteroseptal region.

Comments

Leadless pacemakers at end of life

The projected longevity of Micra leadless PMs is estimated to be comparable to standard transvenous devices, albeit with a programmed pulse width of 0.24 ms (long-term data are still pending).

Reports have shown that leadless PMs can be safely retrieved shortly (months) after implantation,[1] but long-term extraction may be hindered by encapsulation of the device.[2] It has been shown in a study on cadaveric hearts that up to three Micra devices can be implanted without mechanical interaction, but whether this also holds true in the beating heart is unknown.[3]

Contrary to standard devices, for which generator explantation is usually recommended at end of life (due to erratic device behaviour), leadless PMs can be totally inactivated (and therefore abandoned). Finally, leadless PMs do not need to be explanted before cremation.

References

1. Dar T, Akella K, Murtaza G, et al. Comparison of the safety and efficacy of Nanostim and Micra transcatheter leadless pacemaker (LP) extractions: a multicenter experience. *J Interv Card Electrophysiol* 2020; **57**: 133–40.
2. Beurskens NE, Tjong FV, Knops RE. End-of-life management of leadless cardiac pacemaker therapy. *Arrhythm Electrophysiol Rev* 2017; **6**: 129–33.
3. Omdahl P, Eggen MD, Bonner MD, et al. Right ventricular anatomy can accommodate multiple Micra transcatheter pacemakers. *Pacing Clin Electrophysiol* 2016; **39**: 393–7

Introduction to the case

A patient with intermittent third-degree AVB had a leadless Micra AV PM implanted. The device was programmed to VDD mode. Non-tracking of the P-waves was observed on the day following implantation. A real-time recording of the device is shown in Figure 27.1.

Question

Figure 27.1 Real-time recording from the leadless Micra AV PM

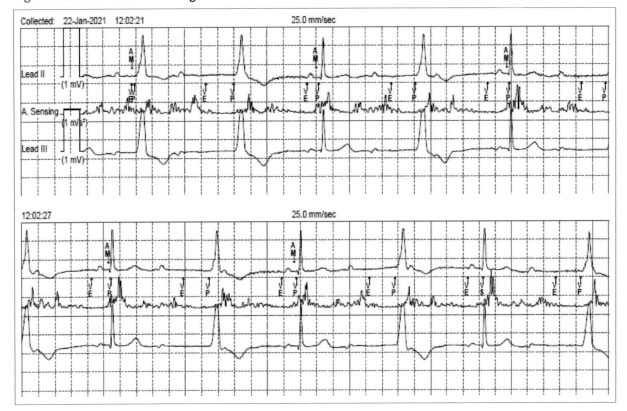

Which modification in the parameters would be most likely to correct the problem?

A Decrease A3 window end

B Decrease A3

D Increase A3 threshold

D Decrease A4 threshold

E Increase A4 threshold

Answer

A Decrease A3 window end

Figure 27.2 Annotated tracing

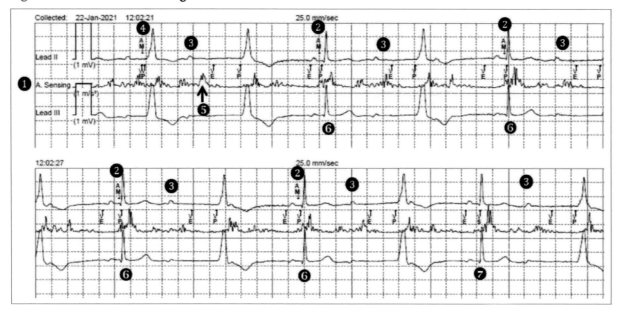

The tracing in Figure 27.2 shows atrial non-tracking due to the A3 window end being too long and covering the A4 signal (corresponding to the P-wave).

❶ The 'A. Sensing' channel displays the signal derived from the accelerometer which the algorithm uses to identify the different mechanical phases of the cardiac cycle (A1–A4).

❷ The marker 'AM' denotes 'Atrial mechanical' or A4, and are appropriately timed after P-waves. This cycle results in AV synchronous pacing. Note the very short programmed delay from AM to VP (nominally programmed at 20 ms).

❸ P-waves which are not detected by the device due to their falling in the PVAB or the A3 window, the end of which is denoted by the 'VE' marker (ventricular event A1–A3 signals).

❹ Delayed AM marker due to late detection of the A4 signal, falling just after the VE marker, explaining the long PR interval.

❺ High-amplitude A7 signal resulting from fusion of the A3 and A4 signals.

❻ Intrinsic AV conduction with pseudo-fusion.

❼ Single cycle with A4 undersensing, resulting in atrial non-tracking. Note the 'VE' marker is before the P-wave, and non-tracking is therefore not explained by the PVAB/A3 window covering the A4 signal. Occasional A4 undersensing can be expected, and this is the not main issue in this case. Note that VS is adequate.

Comments

Leadless VDD pacemakers

Sensing of the atrial signal in the leadless Micra AV PM is based on the signal from the accelerometer. It enables detection of the atrial mechanical systole as well as other events of the cardiac cycle:

- A1: closure of mitral and tricuspid valves.

- A2: closure of aortic and pulmonary valves.

- A3: ventricular diastole, corresponds to E-wave on echocardiography.

- A4: atrial systole, corresponds to A-wave on echocardiography.

The aim of programming is to only sense A4. The PVAB is programmed to cover A1 and A2, and the A3 window to cover A3. The device was programmed with a A3 window end of 875 ms through a auto-setup procedure after implant. A manual atrial mechanical ('MAM') test was performed (Figure 27.3), and the 'A3 window end' was shortened to 650 ms.

Figure 27.3 Manual atrial mechanical (MAM) test. The PVAB should cover the A1 and A2 signals. The A3 threshold (horizontal dotted line in the A3 window) should be *higher* than the A3 signal to avoid A3 oversensing, but not too high as to undersense a signal resulting from fusion of the A3 and A4 signals (= A7 signal). This signal can be observed during tachycardia and corresponds to EA fusion on Doppler echocardiography. The A3 window end should be programmed to cover the entire A3 signal, without encroaching on the A4 signal. The A4 threshold (horizontal line in the A4 window) should be programmed *lower* than the A4 signal. The A4 window ends automatically after detection of AM and the triggered short AV delay

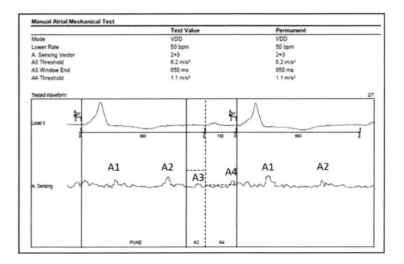

After reprogramming of the 'A3 window end', AV synchronous VDD pacing was established (Figure 27.4).

Figure 27.4 Real-time recording from the leadless Micra AV PM after reprogramming of the 'A3 window end'

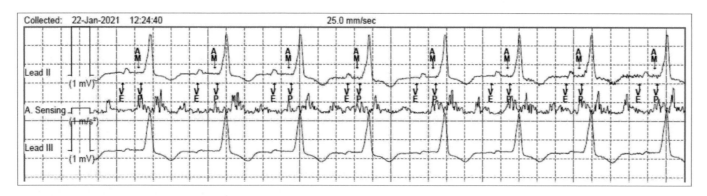

The device is able to track the P-wave up to a rate of 115 bpm (nominal setting of 105 bpm), and clinical studies have shown AV synchronous VDD pacing in 70–90% of the time, depending on patient activity.[1] With faster rates, the sensing algorithm is not able to discern the mechanical atrial contraction, and switches to sensor-driven rate response.

References

1. Steinwender C, Khelae SK, Garweg C, et al. Atrioventricular synchronous pacing using a leadless ventricular pacemaker: results from the MARVEL 2 study. *JACC Clin Electrophysiol* 2020; **6**: 94–106.
2. Garweg C, Khelae SK, Steinwender C, et al. Predictors of atrial mechanical sensing and atrioventricular synchrony with a leadless ventricular pacemaker: Results from the MARVEL 2 Study. *Heart Rhythm* 2020; **17**: 2037–45.

Section Two

ICD

Cases 28–50

Introduction to the case

A patient with mitral valve prolapse and polymorphic VT with syncope was implanted with a dual-chamber ICD. The EGM shown in Figure 28.1 was transmitted by remote monitoring.

Question

Figure 28.1 EGM retrieved by remote monitoring as a non-sustained VT episode

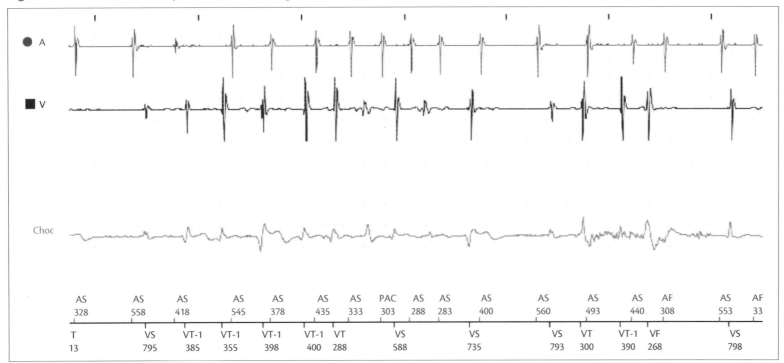

What needs to be done?

A Activate therapy in the VT-1 zone

B Increase ventricular sensitivity (undersensing)

C Reduce ventricular sensitivity (oversensing)

D Revise the ventricular lead (lead fracture)

E None of the above

Answer

E None of the above

Figure 28.2 Annotated tracing

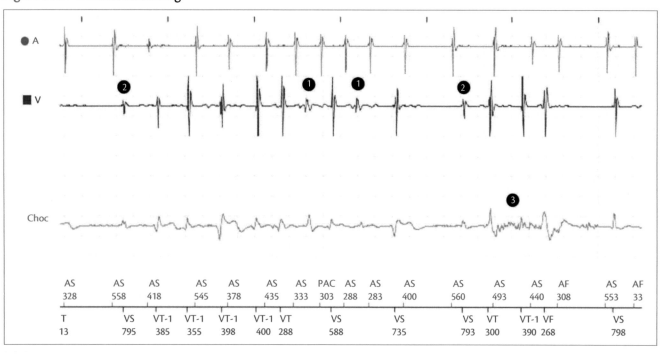

ICD function in this example is normal and does not require any change in programming. The tracing (Figure 28.2) shows a non-sustained episode of arrhythmia with frequent polymorphic PVCs.

❶ These two cycles correspond to PVCs which are undersensed (no corresponding 'VS' marker). Functional undersensing occurs due to the adaptive sensitivity levels and the preceding high-amplitude ventricular premature beats (note the different QRS morphologies in the shock channel).

❷ Conducted sinus beats with relatively low-amplitude ventricular signals, but which are adequately sensed due to the long preceding RR interval which has allowed the sensitivity to adapt to a higher level.

❸ Pectoral myopotentials, visible on the shock channel (can to RV coil), which can be observed under normal circumstances.

Comments

Adaptive implantable cardioverter defibrillator sensitivity levels

Contrary to PMs which may have fixed sensitivity levels set to around 2.0–2.8 mV, ICDs have adaptive sensitivity (Figure 28.3) to avoid T-wave oversensing (TWOS) while allowing the device to detect ventricular tachyarrhythmias with low-amplitude signals. However, many recent PMs also have adaptive sensitivity.

some manufacturers, a plateau is implemented to avoid TWOS. The sensitivity level then increases to the programmed value (usually 0.3–0.8 mV). The increase in sensitivity may be linear (as shown here), in steps, or exponential (Figure 28.4).

Figure 28.4 Different forms of adaptive ICD sensitivity levels (orange, Abbott; red, Boston Scientific; green, Biotronik; blue, Medtronic)

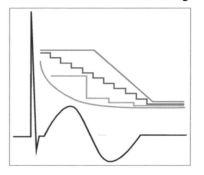

Figure 28.3 Adaptive sensitivity of ICDs. Note how the second cycle is undersensed due to the preceding large electrogram, whereas the third cycle (of identical amplitude as the second cycle) is sensed due to the delay in RR interval

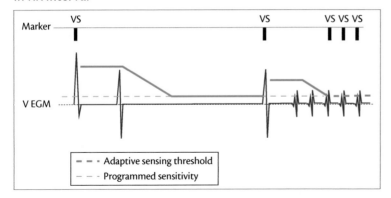

ICD sensing varies among manufacturers but shares some common features. A ventricular blanking period (usually 110–135 ms) avoids R-wave double counting. ICDs only have post-ventricular paced or sensed *blanking* periods. They do not have ventricular *relative refractory* periods, which would defeat the purpose of responding to high-rate ventricular events (contrary to the atrial channel, where relative refractory periods avoid triggering of an AVI). The sensing level usually starts as a percentage (50–75%) of the ventricular EGM amplitude after the refractory period has elapsed (some manufacturers may limit the maximum value). In

Introduction to the case

A 52-year-old female attended the device clinic for follow-up. She had a dual-chamber ICD implanted for secondary prevention due to non-ischaemic dilated cardiomyopathy with sustained VT. The EGM of a recorded episode is shown in Figure 29.1.

Question

Figure 29.1 Recorded arrhythmia episode treated with ATP

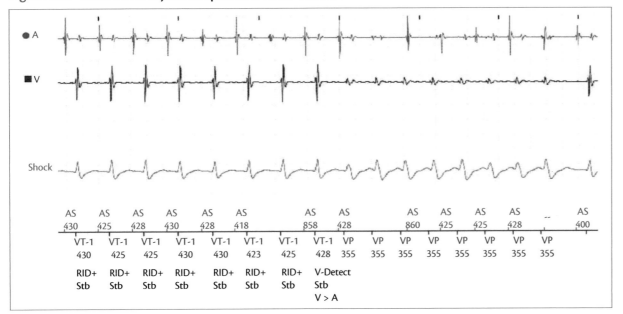

What do you observe?

A Atrial flutter with 2:1 block, inappropriate antitachycardia pacing (ATP)

B Atrial flutter and VT (dual tachycardia)

C AVNRT with inappropriate ATP

D Sinus tachycardia with atrial undersensing leading to inappropriate ATP

E VT with 1:1 VA conduction, treated with ATP

Answer

D Sinus tachycardia with atrial undersensing leading to inappropriate ATP

Figure 29.2 Annotated tracing

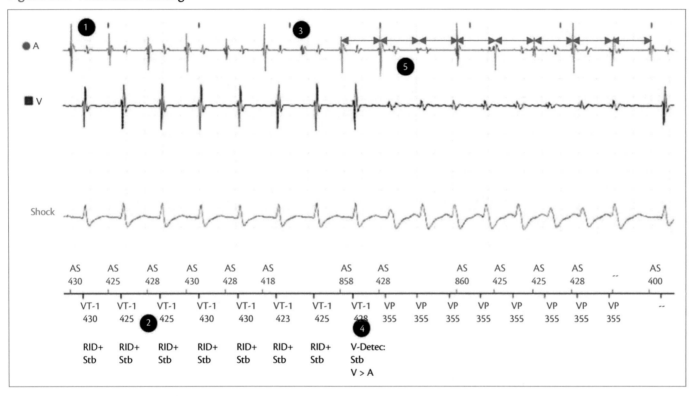

❶ Atrial signals of alternating amplitude, morphology, and cycle lengths (Figure 29.2). The larger signals are sinus rhythm, and the smaller ones FFRWs, which are not sensed as they fall in the PVAB (no corresponding markers).

❷ The rhythm falls in the VT-1 zone. The device determines that the ventricular rate is not greater than the atrial rate (A = V) and then compares a morphology template which matches that seen in normal rhythm. Therapy is initially appropriately withheld (RID+ marker).

❸ Atrial signal of a smaller amplitude, which is undersensed (no corresponding marker).

❹ Due to atrial undersensing, the V > A criterion is fulfilled and VT is detected (V-Detect marker)

❺ Delivery of burst ATP. Far-field ventricular signals can be seen on the atrial EGM. Furthermore, there is retrograde VA block, and sinus rhythm can be seen marching through the tracing, as highlighted by the blue arrows.

Comments

Ventricular tachycardia/supraventricular tachycardia discrimination criteria: V > A, sudden onset and stability

The V > A criterion is usually an over-riding criterion for VT detection in dual-chamber and biventricular ICDs. It may, however, be misled by atrial undersensing due to low-amplitude signals (as in this example), or due to functional undersensing with very short VA intervals and atrial activity falling in the PVAB period (e.g. in case of AVNRT). Some ICDs detect atrial activity in the PVAB (labelled as 'Ab' in the marker channels) for rhythm discrimination (and distinguish this from FFRWs by pattern recognition).

In this Boston Scientific ICD, the device compares an averaged ventricular rate (over 10 beats) versus an average atrial rate (again over 10 beats). If the average ventricular rate is >10 bpm faster than the average atrial rate (V > A marker), VT is detected. Some ICDs compare median rates and would have avoided therapy in this case.

Medtronic dual-chamber and biventricular ICDs have optional sudden onset and stability discrimination criteria. These single-chamber criteria are only applied in the VT zone, but are currently applied first in the decision algorithm. If they diagnose SVT, the rhythm will not undergo any further discrimination (including morphology and dual-chamber criteria such as V > A). This is the reason for which these criteria are by default inactivated in current Medtronic ICDs.

An irregular rhythm is usually associated with SVT. However, VT may also be irregular (but is then usually polymorphic and falls in the VF zone where the regularity criterion is not applied); SVT (including rapidly conducted AF) may be relatively regular.

Unlike sinus tachycardia, VT usually has sudden onset (but so do some SVTs, such as AF). VT may, however, have gradual onset if it is induced at exercise during sinus tachycardia, or if it is suddenly initiated at a rate just below the VT zone with subsequent gradual acceleration (Figure 29.3).

Figure 29.3 Graphical depiction of VT with sudden onset just below the VT zone, and gradual acceleration past the VT limit. This relatively stable VT will be diagnosed as SVT according to the sudden onset criterion

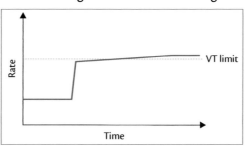

Introduction to the case

A 32-year-old woman attends the device clinic following an episode of palpitations. She had a cardiac resynchronization therapy defibrillator (CRT-D) implanted 2 years previously due to dilated cardiomyopathy with severe LV systolic dysfunction, New York Heart Association (NYHA) class III. She has responded well to CRT and her biventricular pacing percentage is 98%. An arrhythmia episode is shown in Figures 30.1 and 30.2.

Figure 30.1 Details of the arrhythmia episode

Episode Summary	
Initial Type	VF (spontaneous)
Duration	14 sec
A/V Max Rate	Unknown/200 bpm
V. Median	200 bpm (300 ms)
Activity at onset	Rest, Sensor = 59 bpm
Last Therapy	VF Rx 1: Burst + Charging, Successful

Initial VT/VF Detection Withheld By
None

Therapies	Delivered	Charge	Ohms	Energy
Shock aborted because ATP During Charging terminated the rhythm.				
VF Rx 1 Burst	During Charging			
VF Rx 1 Defib	Aborted	5.19 sec		35.0 J
Termination				

Data Collection Setup

	Source	Range
LECG	Can to RVcoil	±2 mV
EGM 1	RVtip to RVring	±8 mV
EGM 2 (Wavelet)	Can to RVcoil	±8 mV
EGM 3	RVtip to RVcoil	±8 mV
Stored (Ventricular)		EGM1 and EGM2
Stored (Atrial)		EGM2 and LECG
Pre-arrhythmia EGM		Off

Wavelet Measurements Prior to Initial VT/VF Detecion

Wavelet Result: VT/VF
Template Status: OK

–8.	No Match	61%
–7.	No Match	58%
–6.	No Match	68%
–5.	No Match	65%
–4.	No Match	58%
–3.	No Match	61%
–2.	No Match	61%
–1.	No Match	58%
0.	Detection	

Parameter Settings		Initial	Redetect	V. Interval (Rate)
VF	On	30/40	12/16	320 ms (188 bpm)
FVT	Off			
VT	Off	16	12	
Monitor	Off	32		

PR Logic/Wavelet	
AF/Afl	On
Sinus Tach	On
Other 1:1 SVTs	Off
Wavelet	On, Match = 70%
Template	12-May-2016, Auto = Off
SVT V. Limit	260 ms

Other Enhancements	
Stability	Off
Onset	Off
High Rate Timeout	
VF Zone Only	Off
TWave	On
RV Lead Noise	On + Timeout
Timeout	0.75 min

Type	ATP Seq	Shocks	Success	ID#	Date	Time hh:mm	Duration hh:mm:ss	Avg bpm A/V	Max bpm A/V	Activity at Onset
VF	1		Yes	6	18-Jun-2016	09:38	:14	200/200	- - -/200	Rest

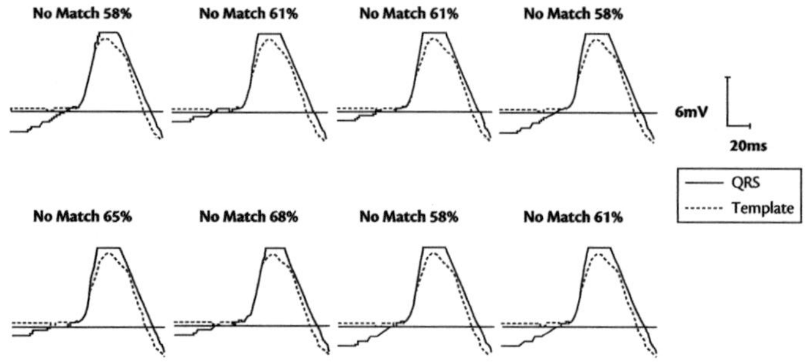

Question

Figure 30.2 EGM of the arrhythmia episode

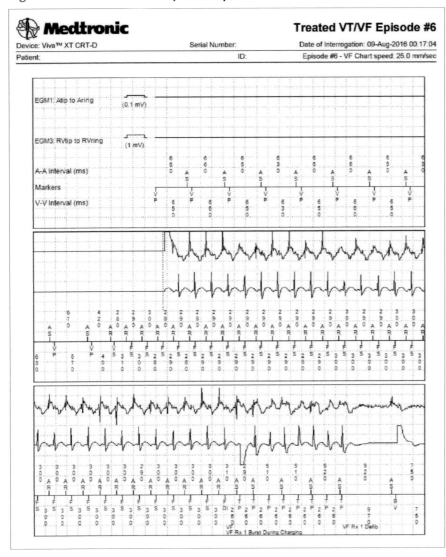

What would be the best way to reduce the risk of further therapy due to this arrhythmia?

A Commence amiodarone

B Enable 'Other 1:1 SVTs' criterion

C Increase SVT limit rate

D Modify morphology discrimination algorithm settings

E Prolong the number of intervals to detection (NID)

Answer

D Modify morphology discrimination algorithm settings

Figure 30.3 Marker channel, device settings, and wavelet diagnostics

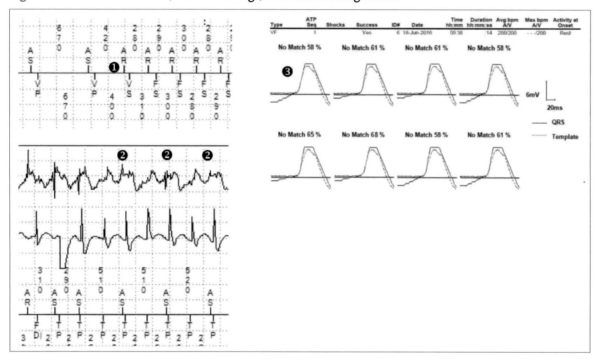

❶ Onset of arrhythmia with a premature atrial contraction (Figure 30.3), indicative that the arrhythmia is likely to be supraventricular in origin. VT which initiated nearly simultaneously with the atrial premature contraction is possible, but unlikely. There is 1:1 association between the atrial and ventricular signals throughout the tachycardia, with little variation in the AV and VA intervals. The tachycardia cycle length (300 ms) is longer than the SVT limit (260 ms). Therefore, discrimination algorithms are already applied and increasing the SVT limit rate would not help. The VA interval here is too long for the 'Other 1:1 SVTs' criterion to withhold therapy. The feature is, however, useful to discriminate between ventricular tachyarrhythmias and rhythms that result in closely coupled atrial and ventricular depolarizations (such as AVNRT). It should, however, only be turned on once the atrial lead has stabilized (otherwise lead dislodgement to the ventricle will result in withholding of therapy for true VT). Increasing the NID would simply delay inevitable therapy.

❷ Antitachycardia burst pacing at 260 ms cycle length inducing 2:1 VA block (AA intervals 510–520 ms) with interruption of the tachycardia. It is unclear if there was reset of atrial activity by the first ATP cycle (slightly shorted AA interval of 290 ms), but the differential diagnosis is a nodal tachycardia (atypical AVNRT) or AT which terminated spontaneously during the burst.

❸ Morphology template with signal clipping. There seems to be a close match between the arrhythmia QRS and the stored template. Had the signal not been clipped, it would almost certainly have matched and therapy would have been withheld. The morphology settings should be modified to avoid clipping by increasing the signal range (currently set to ±8 mV).

Comments

Morphology discrimination algorithm

Morphology discrimination relies on the fact that the majority of SVTs have no change in QRS morphology. The device collects a template, typically taken from a far-field EGM of RV coil to can. During detection, the device analyses the ventricular EGM and compares it to the stored EGM during sinus rhythm, completing a match score. The default match score varies from manufacturer to manufacturer, but is typically in the range of 70–94%. Typically, if 3/10 beats are a 'match', the device will withhold therapy. QRS morphology analysis forms a part of nearly all ICDs used in clinical practice, whether single-lead defibrillators, dual-chamber defibrillators, or CRT-Ds.

Given that inappropriate therapy was delivered due to signal clipping, the easiest way to resolve this problem would be to increase the channel range. The template waveform should only fill roughly two-thirds of the range window to accommodate for increase in EGM amplitude during tachycardia. The percentage match should be evaluated during setup on a beat-to-beat basis. If matching is very variable, this could be due to the range being too large (i.e. the template insufficiently fills the window), or due to a suboptimal vector. The vector can usually be reprogrammed, but there may be interlock with lead integrity algorithms (which may require to be inactivated). In this respect, dual-coil ICD leads are useful, as they provide additional vector options. The template is automatically updated on a periodic basis in most devices.

Morphology discrimination algorithms are ineffective in case of rate-dependent aberrancy. An option in this instance is to collect the template with QRS aberrancy (e.g. during rapid AP or during exercise in a patient with AF), and inactivate the auto-update function.

Introduction to the case

A patient with dilated cardiomyopathy with a history of sustained VT had a dual-chamber ICD implanted at another centre for secondary prevention. Device settings are shown in Figure 31.1. He consulted after having experienced a shock. The EGM retrieved from the device memory is shown in Figure 31.2.

Figure 31.1 Device tachycardia detection and therapy settings

	VT	VF
Detection Criteria	160 min–1/375 ms 30 intervals	200 min–1/300 ms 30 intervals
SVT Discrimination	On	
Therapy	ATP x3 ATP x3 36.0 J/845 V 40.0 J/890 V x2	ATP x1 30.0 J/771 V 40.0 J/890 V 40.0 J/890 V x4
VT Therapy Timeout	Off	

SVT Discrimination

SVT Discrimination	Dual Chamber
SVT Discrimination Timeout	Off
SVT Upper Limit	Same as VF

Rate Branch	Additional Discriminators				Diagnosis
AF/A Flutter V < A	**Morphology** Morphology Match Auto Update	On 60%, 7 of 12 1 day	**Interval Stability** Interval Stability Stability Delta AV Association Delta Window Size	On W/AVA 40 ms 60 ms 12 intervals	If All of the criteria in this rate branch indicate VT, deliver therapy.
Sinus Tach V = A: On AV Interval Delta: 60 ms	**Morphology** Morphology Match Auto Update	On 60%, 7 of 12 1 day	**Sudden Onset** Sudden Onset Onset Delta	On 20%	If All of the criteria in this rate branch indicate VT, deliver therapy.
VT/VF V > A					If Ventricular Rate is greater than the Atrial Rate, deliver therapy.

Question

Figure 31.2 EGM retrieved from the device memory

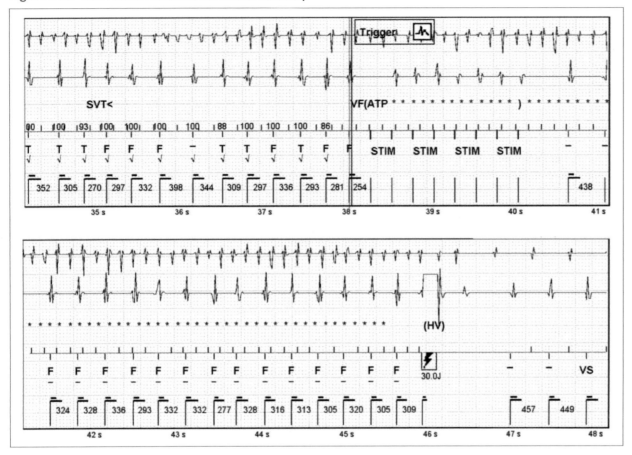

Why is a shock delivered?

A Appropriate shock for VT

B Appropriate shock for dual tachycardia

C Misdiagnosis due to morphology discrimination

D No discrimination algorithms are applied

E SVT discrimination timeout

Answer

D No discrimination algorithms are applied

Figure 31.3 Annotated tracing

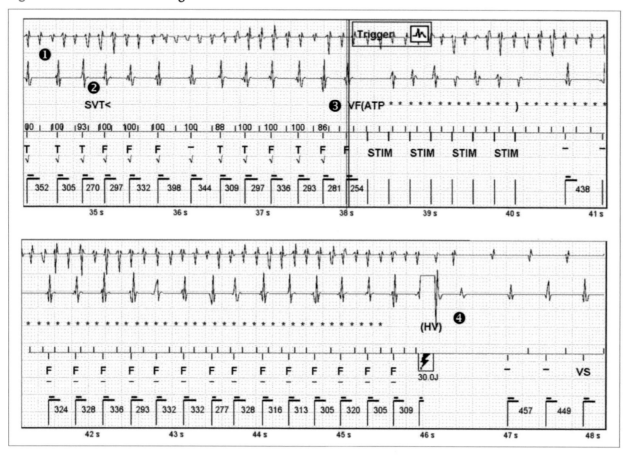

Rapidly conducted AF falling in the VF zone results in an inappropriate shock with cardioversion to sinus rhythm (Figure 31.3).

❶ AF with rapid irregular AV conduction. All ventricular cycles are above the 60% morphology match threshold (labelled '✓')

❷ The VT counters are filled but SVT is diagnosed due to correct discrimination (morphology and interval stability). In this device, all arrhythmia counters ('bins') are reset to 0 at this point.

❸ This device only requires six intervals to redetect an arrhythmia (for initial detection, 30 intervals are required, as shown in Figure 31.1). The VF counters are filled at this point, with diagnosis of VF. As SVT discriminators are not applied in the VF zone in this device, therapy is delivered.

❹ The 30 J shock cardioverts the AF back to sinus rhythm.

The SVT discriminator timeout feature had been inactivated (Figure 31.1).

Comments

Supraventricular tachycardia discriminators and arrhythmia zones

Most ICD manufacturers only have SVT discriminators programmed in VT zones (and not VF zones)—see Figure 31.4, but in some devices (e.g. Medtronic) they can be programmed to extend to within the VF zone.

Figure 31.4 VT zones and SVT discriminators of ICDs. Some ICDs have discriminators which can be programmed to extend to within the VF zone (dotted area)

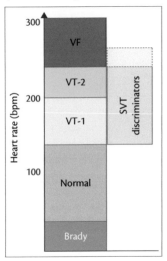

SVT discriminators should be routinely activated in all patients, an exception being those with complete AVB. In the present case, device settings were changed to increase the VF zone to 240 bpm and a VT-2 zone from 187–240 bpm was added (where SVT discriminators are applied). The morphology cut-off in this generation of ICDs was nominally set at 60% and was based on a near-field template (current technology used a far-field template with a cut-off of 90%).

It is important to note that SVT discriminators mainly affect initial rhythm discrimination of an episode. They are mostly not applied upon *redetection* of an arrhythmia after first failed therapy (ATP or shock) due to risk of alteration in the properties of the arrhythmia after therapy (e.g. change in EGM morphology of an SVT or cycle length irregularity of a VT).

Recommended settings for ICD programming from all major manufacturers have been published and are useful as a guide for daily practice.[1]

Reference

1. Stiles MK, Fauchier L, Morillo CA, Wilkoff BL. 2019 HRS/EHRA/APHRS/LAHRS focused update to 2015 expert consensus statement on optimal implantable cardioverter-defibrillator programming and testing. *Europace* 2019; **21**: 1442–3.

Introduction to the case

A 34-year-old man is brought to the emergency room via ambulance reporting multiple conscious shocks from his device. He had a VVI ICD implanted 3 years previously for dilated cardiomyopathy with severe LV systolic dysfunction and haemodynamically unstable VT. His device settings and scatter plot are shown in Figure 32.1, and one of the arrhythmia episodes is shown in Figure 32.2.

Figure 32.1 Device settings and scatter plot

Medtronic **Parameters**

Device: Visia AF MRI™ XT VR Serial Number: Date of Interrogation: 26-Mar-2018 10:49:48

Patient: ID: Physician:

VT/VF Detection

		V. Interval (Rate)	Initial	Redetect
VF	On	320 ms (188 bpm)	30/40	12/16
FVT	OFF			
VT	OFF	360 ms (167 bpm)	16	12
Monitor	Off	450 ms (133 bpm)	32	

Wavelet		Other Enhancements		Sensitivity	
Wavelet	On	Stability	Off	RV	0.30 mV
Template	26-Jan-2018	Onset	Off		
Match Threshold	70 %	High Rate Timeout			
Auto Collection	Off	VF Zone Only	Off		
SVT V. Limit	260 ms	TWave	On		
		RV Lead Noise	On+Timeout		
		Timeout	0.75 min		

VF Therapies	Rx1	Rx2	Rx3	Rx4	Rx5	Rx6
VF Therapy Status	On	On	On	On	On	On
Energy	35 J	35 J	35 J	35 J	35 J	35 J
Pathway	B>AX*	B>AX*	B>AX*	B>AX*	AX>B*	B>AX*

* SVC Coil Off

ATP During Charging

Deliver ATP if last 8 R-R >= 240 ms, Burst, Pulses = 8, R-S1 = 88 %, Decrement = 10 ms

ChargeSaver = On(1 episodes), SmartMode = On

FVT Therapies	Rx1	Rx2	Rx3	Rx4	Rx5	Rx6
FVT Therapy Status	Off	Off	Off	Off	Off	Off

VT Therapies	Rx1	Rx2	Rx3	Rx4	Rx5	Rx6
VT Therapy Status	Off	Off	Off	Off	Off	Off

Shared V. ATP		Shared V. Therapies	
V-V Minimum ATP Interval	200 ms	Active Can/SVC Coil	SVC Off
V. Amplitude	8 V	Progressive Episode Therapies	Off
V. Pulse Width	1.5 ms	Confirmation+	On
V. Pace Blanking	240 ms		

Medtronic **Treated VT/VF Episode #1614**

Device: Visia AF MRI™ XT VR Serial Number: Date of Interrogation: 26-Mar-2018 10:49:48

Patient: ID: Physician:

Type	ATP Seq	Shocks	Success	ID#	Date	Time hh:mm	Duration hh:mm:ss	Avg bpm V	Max bpm V	Activity at Onset
VF	0	6	No	1614	28-Feb-2018	03:39	:21:16	240	286	Rest

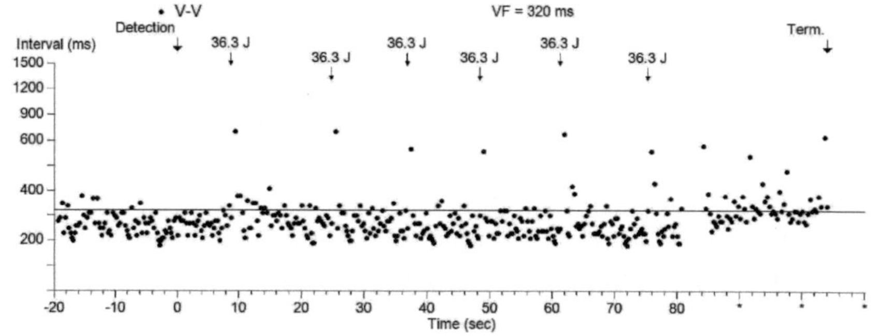

Question

Figure 32.2 Arrhythmia episode

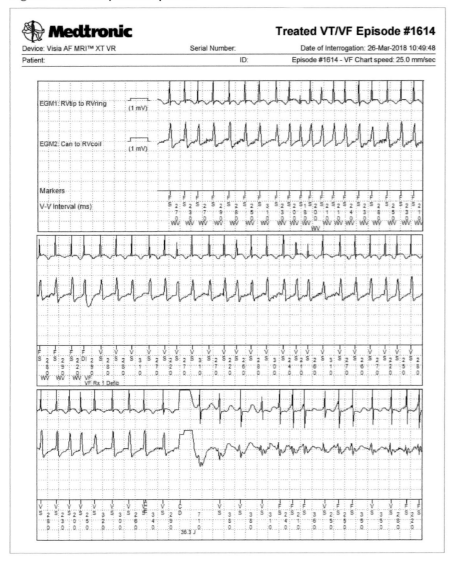

Which of the following measures will reliably avoid further shocks in this patient?

A Enable fast VT zone in order to deliver further cycles of ATP

B Enable 'onset' for SVT discrimination

C Enable 'stability' for SVT discrimination

D Increase SVT limit

E None of the above

Answer

E None of the above

Figure 32.3 Annotated EGM

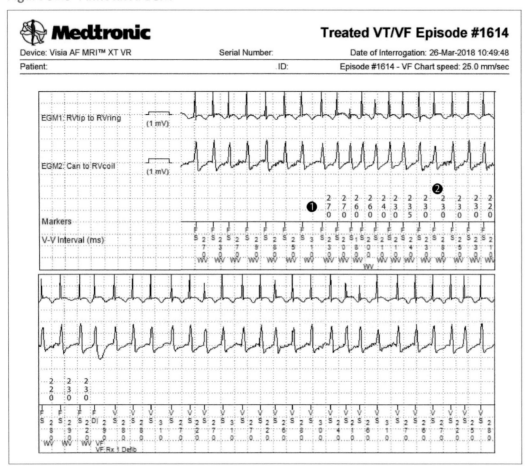

The patient has inappropriate shocks due to very rapidly conducted AF (Figure 32.3).

❶ This is a VR ICD which is using morphology (Wavelet) as the only SVT discriminator as per current recommendations. Therapy is initially withheld by the algorithm ('WV' marker). The arrhythmia shows marked cycle variability indicating that the arrhythmia is likely to be AF. The sudden onset and stability criteria are only active in VT zones, and this patient only has a VF zone programmed. Even if a fast VT zone were programmed, the arrhythmia is so rapidly conducted that it is likely to fall in the VF zone.

❷ The SVT limit is programmed to 260 ms, but the arrhythmia cycles are frequently shorter (i.e. faster) than this limit. Even increasing the SVT limit to the shortest programmed cycle length of 240 ms would not solve the problem.

Comments

Supraventricular tachycardia limit

As seen in Case 31, all defibrillators have a limit at which SVT discriminators can be applied. For all ICD manufacturers apart from Medtronic, SVT discriminators are only applicable in the VT zones. Medtronic ICDs allow extension of the SVT discriminators in the VF zone to withhold therapy in case of rapidly conducted arrhythmias. The default setting is 260 ms, with the shortest programmable limit (fastest rate) of 240 ms (250 bpm).

The decision to withhold therapy is always re-evaluated during tachycardia, so as not to miss arrhythmias such as exercise-induced VT and VT/VF during episodes of rapidly conducted AF. In Medtronic devices, the median ventricular rate is calculated over the preceding 12 beats. If the median rate exceeds the programmed SVT limit, this indicates that discrimination should no longer be applied and a 'transition counter' begins. The counter decreases from 10 each time the median rate is above the SVT limit, and once it reaches 0, there is enough evidence that the arrhythmia has changed and the discriminators are no longer applied (such as in the present example).

The best options to avoid inappropriate therapy in this patient would be to increase rate-slowing drugs (beta-blockers) to slow ventricular response in case of recurrent AF, perform pulmonary vein isolation, and treat with amiodarone if necessary. If these measures fail, an 'ablate and pace' strategy (with either conduction system pacing or biventricular pacing) may be necessary to avoid inappropriate shocks.

In patients with permanent complete AVB, SVT discriminators should be inactivated as there will no longer be conducted supraventricular arrhythmias (but the RV lead noise and TWOS algorithms should be left on).

Introduction to the case

A patient with ischaemic heart disease and a history of sustained VT had been implanted 3 days ago with a dual-chamber ICD. He consulted for malaise with two shocks. Device parameters are shown in Table 33.1. The EGM of the episode is shown in Figure 33.1.

Table 33.1 Device parameters

Pacing mode	AAI/DDD 40 bpm
Monitor zone (133–167 bpm)	No therapy (NID 32)
Slow VT zone	167–188 bpm (NID 20; redetection 12)
Fast VT zone	188–250 bpm (30/40; redetection 12/16)
VF zone	>250 bpm (30/40; redetection 12/16)
SVT discriminators (SVT limit 260 ms)	Morphology (wavelet): on Stability: off Sudden onset: monitor Dual-chamber discriminators: AT/AF on Sinus tachycardia: on Other 1:1 SVT: off

Question

Figure 33.1 EGM retrieved from the device memory

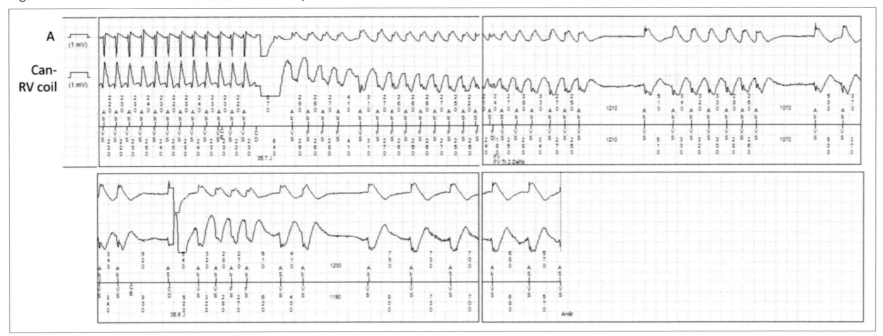

What do you observe?

A AVNRT

B Asynchronous shocks

C HBP lead connected to the atrial port

D Lead dislodgment

E Non-committed second shock

Answer

D Lead dislodgment

Figure 33.2 Annotated tracing

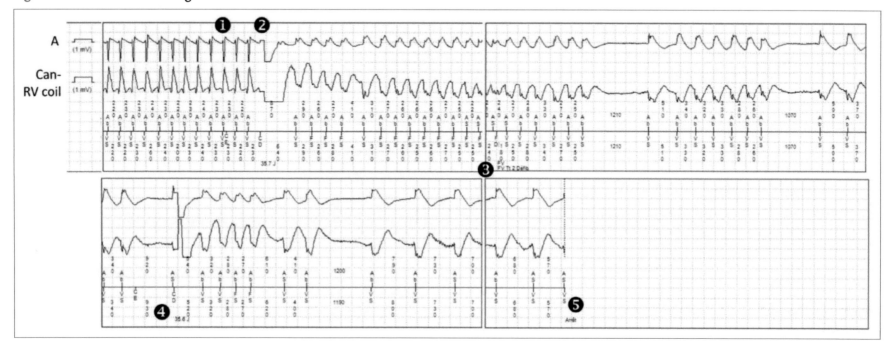

❶ A monomorphic VT falling within the VF zone and at a shorter cycle length than the SVT discriminators is shown in Figure 33.2 at the end of capacitor charge (CE marker). Atrial and ventricular events are synchronous *throughout* the entire tracing (i.e. also after end of the tachycardia), which indicates that the atrial lead has dislodged to the ventricle rather than the initial arrhythmia being AVNRT. Note also that the amplitude of the signals in the atrial channel is about 10 mV, which indicates ventricular rather than atrial potentials. The observation would be compatible with a lead implanted on the His bundle or LBB area, but the dual-chamber discriminators would have all been inactivated in this instance.

❷ At the end of capacitor charge (CE marker), the arrhythmia is confirmed by 2/5 fast intervals (230 and 220 ms) and the charge is delivered (CD marker), synchronized to an

R wave (which explains the slight delay to shock delivery after confirmation). This shock induces non-sustained polymorphic VT.

❸ *Redetection* of the arrhythmia after therapy delivery occurs after 12 fast intervals (12/16 programmed criterion), initiating a new capacitor charge.

❹ At the end of capacitor charge, a *committed* second shock is delivered and induces non-sustained polymorphic VT. Note again the slight delay to shock delivery, as the device attempts to synchronize the shock to an R-wave, and delivers a shock after 900 ms have passed without a VS.

❺ The episode ends after detection of eight consecutive cycles falling outside the tachycardia zone.

Comments

Different aspects of implantable cardioverter defibrillator function

In this case, the atrial lead was repositioned, the single-coil ICD lead was replaced by a dual-coil lead, and defibrillation testing was performed successfully. It is possible that the dislodged atrial lead in the ventricle had a proarrhythmic effect.

This example illustrates why it is important to inactivate 1:1 SVT discriminators until the atrial lead has stabilized, as a true VT may be classified as a junctional tachycardia. Atrial events falling in the PVAB are detected as atrial blanked events ('Ab' marker in this case). These events are not used for pacing functions (e.g. mode switching in case of AT/AF), but for VT/SVT rhythm discrimination. A short and constant VS–Ab interval indicates junctional tachycardia such as AVNRT. The VT in this example was faster than the SVT discrimination limit and would have been appropriately detected even if the 1:1 SVT discriminator had been activated.

First shocks are always nominally *non-committed* at the end of capacitor charge (requiring in this device at least 2/5 fast intervals for *confirmation* of arrhythmia before the shock is delivered). Second and consecutive shocks in the VF zone are always *committed* (i.e. there is no confirmation of persistence of ventricular arrhythmia at the end of capacitor charge and before shock delivery) as reduction in signal amplitude during the delay may lead to undersensing of ventricular arrhythmia. Second and consecutive shocks may however be non-committed in fast VT and VT zones. SVT discriminators are usually not applied for *redetection* of arrhythmias (i.e. diagnosis of persistence of ventricular arrhythmia after therapy delivery) due to the propensity to alter the arrhythmia (e.g. irregular VT induced by ATP or change in signal morphology after a shock). In this device, the stability criterion is, however, applied for redetection in the VT zone.

Introduction to the case

A patient with a DDD ICD presented for follow-up. He complained of palpitations and dizziness. The EGM of an episode of arrhythmia is shown in Figure 34.1.

Question

Figure 34.1 EGM of episode retrieved from the ICD memory

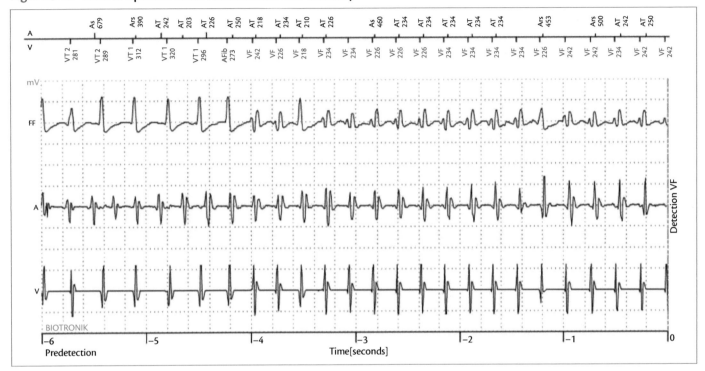

What do you observe?

A Acceleration of atrial flutter to 1:1 AV conduction

B Acceleration of VT

C Dual tachycardia

D Sinus tachycardia accelerating to VT

E VF

Answer

C Dual tachycardia

Figure 34.2 Annotated EGM

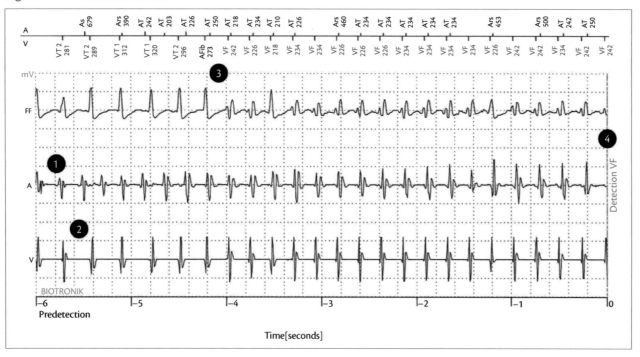

❶ AT/atrial flutter (Figure 34.2), with intermittent undersensing (no AS/ARS markers) due to cross-chamber blanking (atrial activity falling in the PVAB) and due to low amplitude (e.g. fourth atrial cycle).

❷ Rapid conduction of the AT/atrial flutter, falling in the fast (VT2) and slow (VT1) zones.

❸ Increase in ventricular rate and change in near- and far-field EGM, suggestive of VT.

❹ After 18 cycles, detection of VF (indicating that the VF detection criterion was set at 18/24).

Comments

Dual tachycardias

Coexisting SVT and VTs are not unusual, and one arrhythmia may trigger the other. Careful analysis of the onset, A:V relationship, morphology, regularity, and termination, help clarify whether one is dealing with a rapidly conducted SVT or dual tachycardia.

In this case, ATP was delivered, with interruption of the VT but triggering of AF, probably due to retrograde conduction of the ATP sequence (Figure 34.3).

Figure 34.3 Sequel to Figure 34.1. Delivery of ATP with interruption of the VT but triggering of AF (probably due to retrograde conduction)

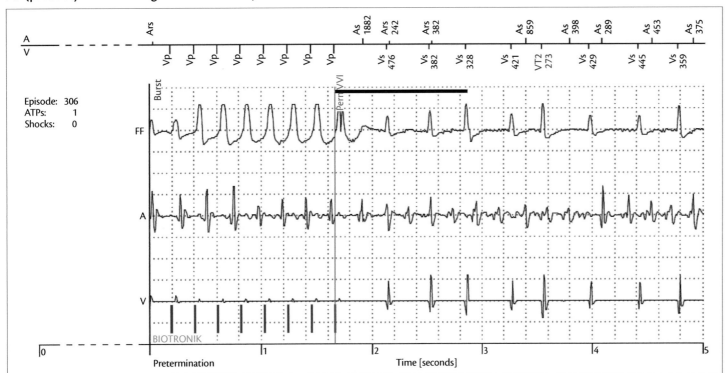

Introduction to the case

A 35-year-old patient with dilated cardiomyopathy implanted with a CRT-D presented for follow-up. He complained of occasional palpitations. An arrhythmic episode retrieved from the device memory is shown in Figure 35.1.

Question

Figure 35.1 Recorded EGM

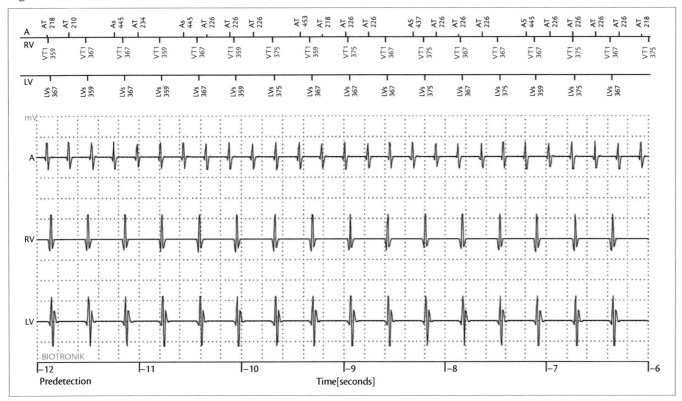

What is your diagnosis?

A AF

B AT/atrial flutter with conduction to the ventricles

C AVNRT

D Atrioventricular reentrant tachycardia (AVRT)

E Dual tachycardia

Answer

E Dual tachycardia

Figure 35.2 Annotated EGM

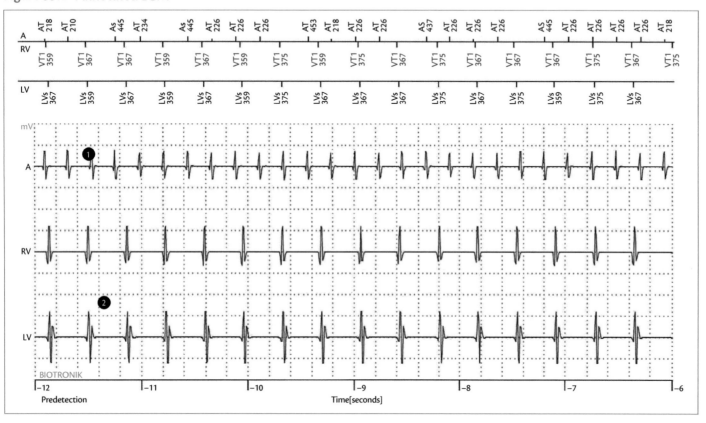

The tracing in Figure 35.2 shows AT/atrial flutter with concomitant VT (i.e. dual tachycardia).

❶ The atrial channel shows a regular activity at a cycle length of 210–226 ms (AF would have been more irregular) with occasional functional undersensing (atrial event falling in the PVAB). The A:V ratio is >1, ruling out AVRT.

❷ Monomorphic regular ventricular cycles at 359–375 ms, with simultaneous RV and LV activation (with possibly a circuit near the interventricular septum). Note that there is no relation between atrial and ventricular activation (AV dissociation), which points against conducted SVT. The irregular VA intervals point against AVNRT with 2:1 AVB.

Comments

A > V tachycardia

The majority of A > V tachycardias which are recorded in VT zones are supraventricular arrhythmias with rapid ventricular conduction. Ventricular rate may be relatively regular in case of very rapidly conducted AF, or in case of 2:1 response of conducted AT/atrial flutter. In the latter case, there is a clear AV relationship. Ventricular response may also be irregular due to a Wenckebach conduction.

On occasions, AVNRT may be observed with 2:1 AVB,[1] which is present in up to 10% of induced AVNRT and due to functional infranodal block.[2] However, the VA intervals in these instances is constant (Figure 35.3)

Figure 35.3 Episode of AVNRT with 2:1 AVB transitioning to 1:1 conduction after a ventricular premature beat (*). Note the constant VA intervals throughout, as well as aberrancy in QRS morphology (visible in the shock channel) with 1:1 conduction

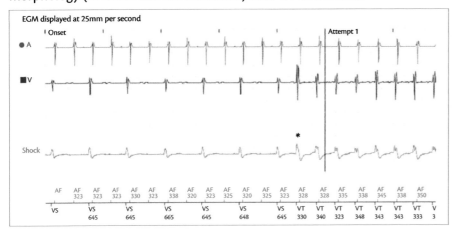

Reproduced from Burri H. A 2:1 Atrioventricular Tachycardia Recorded by an Implantable Cardioverter Defibrillator: What Is the Mechanism? *J Cardiovasc Electrophysiol.* 2016 Dec;27(12):1492–1494. doi: 10.1111/jce.13056 with permission from John Wiley and Sons

Reference

1. Burri H. A 2:1 atrioventricular tachycardia recorded by an implantable cardioverter defibrillator: what is the mechanism? *J Cardiovasc Electrophysiol* 2016; **27**: 1492–4.
2. Man KC, Brinkman K, Bogun F, et al. 2:1 atrioventricular block during atrioventricular node reentrant tachycardia. *J Am Coll Cardiol* 1996; **28**: 1770–4.

Introduction to the case

A patient with arrhythmogenic RV dysplasia and a VVI ICD implanted 5 years ago consulted the outpatient clinic after syncope. Device interrogation revealed the tracing shown in Figure 36.1.

Question

Figure 36.1 EGM retrieved from the device memory

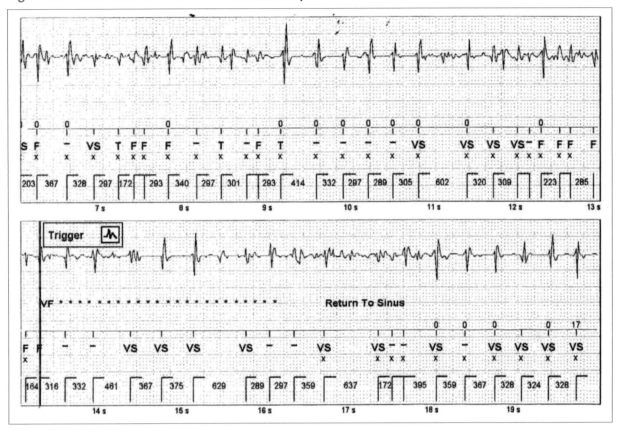

What is your diagnosis?

A AF leading to inappropriate VF detection

B Electromagnetic interference (EMI)

C Lead fracture

D Lead displaced to the atrium

E VF

Answer

E VF

Figure 36.2 Annotated EGM

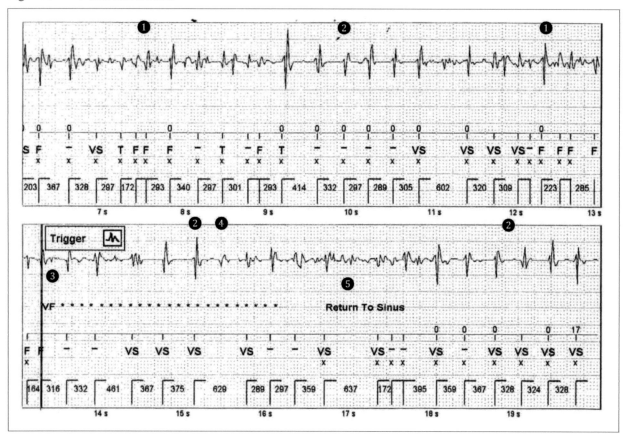

❶ Detection of polymorphic R-waves corresponding to VF (Figure 36.2). This older device did not store far-field EGMs, which would have been useful to more easily identify VF.

❷ Transient organization of the VF into polymorphic VT (note the morphology discrimination algorithm indicating 0% match). The RR intervals on occasion fall below the VT detection rate (VS markers).

❸ VF criteria are met and charging begins.

❹ Underdetection of low-amplitude R waves after a high-amplitude R wave. This is due to dynamic sensitivity (see Case 28).

❺ Repeated undersensing of low-amplitude VF, with false 'Return to Sinus' with abortion of therapy. The arrhythmia, however, subsequently terminated spontaneously.

Comments

Undersensing of ventricular fibrillation

This case illustrates how VF may on rare occasions revert spontaneously without defibrillation.

Undersensing of VF is a dreaded and potentially lethal event, which may be due to low EGM amplitude, deviation from recommended programming, or adhesion to guidelines extrapolated from evidence obtained using another manufacturer's ICDs with different sensing and detection features.[1] Interaction of manufacturer-specific features with generic programming include different counting methods to satisfy arrhythmia detection/duration/termination, different SVT discriminating algorithms, and different enhancements to minimize TWOS (such as a delay to increase sensitivity level, or low-frequency attenuation filters which may reduce the amplitude of VF EGMs[2]).

Ultimately, the dilemma is to balance the risks of failure to treat VF with the risks of inappropriate therapies. In the present case, sensitivity of the ventricular channel was increased, and defibrillation testing performed to evaluate adequate device function.

References

1. Thøgersen AM, Larsen JM, Johansen JB, Abedin M, Swerdlow CD. Failure to treat life-threatening ventricular tachyarrhythmias in contemporary implantable cardioverter-defibrillators: implications for strategic programming. *Circ Arrhythm Electrophysiol* 2017; **10**: e005305.
2. Swerdlow CD, Asirvatham SJ, Ellenbogen KA, Friedman PA. Troubleshooting implanted cardioverter defibrillator sensing problems I. *Circ Arrhythm Electrophysiol* 2014; 7: 1237–61.

Introduction to the case

The tracing shown in Figure 37.1 was sent by remote monitoring in a patient with a DDD ICD which had been implanted 9 years ago. Electrical parameters were normal, except for battery voltage which was reaching elective replacement indicator (ERI).

Question

Figure 37.1 EGM transmitted by remote monitoring as a 'periodic recording' from a dual-chamber ICD

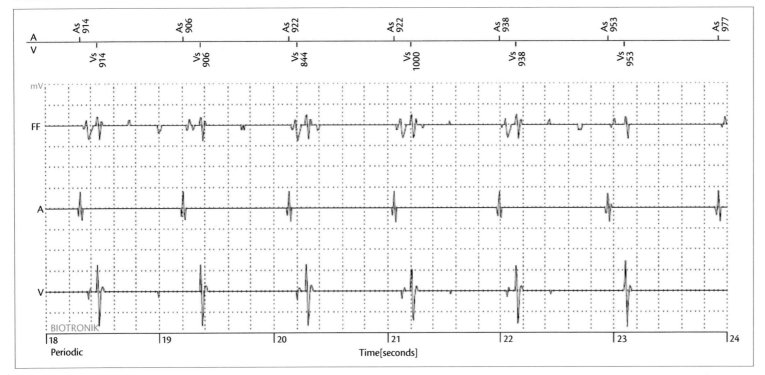

What is the most likely diagnosis?

A Circuit problem

B Diaphragmatic myopotentials

C EMI

D Lead fracture

E Pectoral myopotentials

Answer

D Lead fracture

Figure 37.2 Annotated EGM

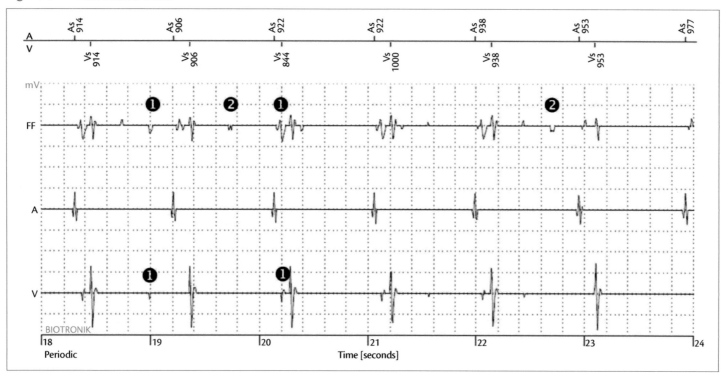

The artefacts in Figure 37.2 are subtle indications of ventricular lead fracture.

❶ Noise appearing simultaneously in the near-field (RV tip to ring) and far-field (can to RV coil) EGM channels. Some of the artefacts are synchronous with the cardiac cycles, suggesting that the site of fracture may be intracardiac. The artefacts are not detected by the device (no corresponding markers). Note absence of noise on the atrial channel, speaking against EMI.

❷ Noise on the far-field ventricular channel only. This may be due to artefacts generated only by RV coil fracture, or due to sampling on the near-field ventricular channel missing these signals, or due to very low-amplitude signals not reaching the threshold to be displayed (Zeroband feature, designed to compress the signal—see explanation of Case 66).

Comments

Lead fracture

Lead fracture may manifest itself by generation of artefacts (which may be recorded as short RR intervals, high-rate episodes, or result in inappropriate shocks), increasing threshold, and/or abnormal lead impedance. It is important to carefully review atrial or ventricular high-rate episodes, as these may reveal fracture potentials. Periodic EGM transmissions by remote monitoring can also provide valuable indices (as illustrated by the present case). Short detected RR intervals may also trigger remote monitoring alerts if certain criteria are fulfilled.

Artefacts are usually of large amplitude and erratic, but may be occasionally of low amplitude or rhythmed by cardiac cycles if they are located within the heart (as in the present case). If the fracture is due to subclavian crush or friction with the generator, noise may be provoked by arm movement or manipulation of the subclavian region or the pocket and identified by viewing the real-time EGM.

Lead impedance may be normal, due to the sampling during good conductor contact. Therefore, normal lead impedance cannot rule out lead fracture.

Some manufacturers (currently Abbott and Medtronic) have specific noise detection algorithms which rely upon detection of high-rate signals, variations in lead impedance and/or comparison of near-field and far-field electrograms. Remote monitoring is useful for early detection of lead fracture.

In the present case, lead fracture was not recognized, and the patient underwent generator change. Detection of ventricular high-rate episodes subsequently revealed clear indices of lead fracture in the ventricular channel (Figure 37.3), and the patient underwent lead revision.

Figure 37.3 Fracture potentials detected as a non-sustained ventricular high-rate episode

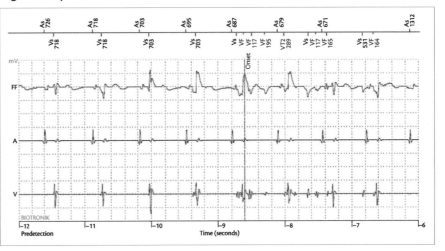

Introduction to the case

A patient with a CRT-D was seen at follow-up. The patient had no complaints. Biventricular pacing was delivered in 96% of the time, with 4% VS events. The tracing shown in Figure 38.1 was retrieved from the device memory as a 'ventricular oversensing' event.

Question

Figure 38.1 Event retrieved from the device memory

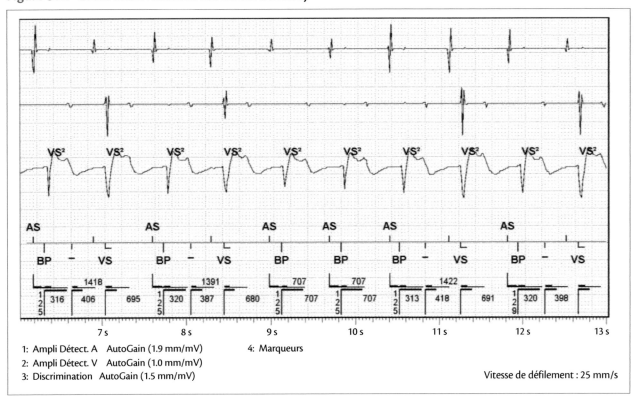

1: Ampli Détect. A   AutoGain (1.9 mm/mV)   4: Marqueurs
2: Ampli Détect. V   AutoGain (1.0 mm/mV)
3: Discrimination   AutoGain (1.5 mm/mV)   Vitesse de défilement : 25 mm/s

What do you observe?

A Atrial undersensing

B R-wave double counting

C TWOS

D Ventricular premature beats

E None of the above

Answer

c TWOS

Figure 38.2 Annotated tracing

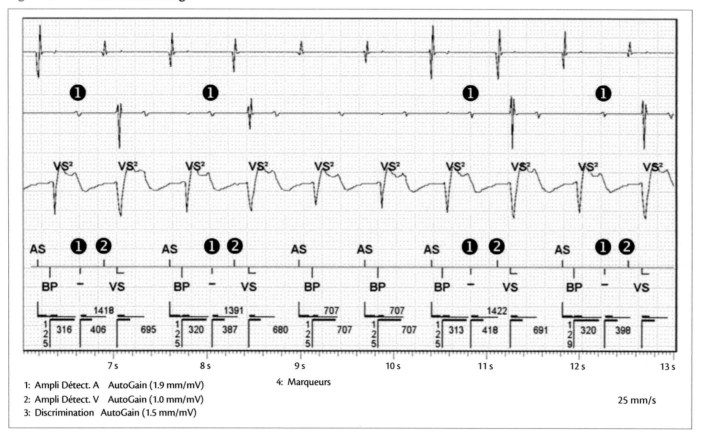

1: Ampli Détect. A   AutoGain (1.9 mm/mV)
2: Ampli Détect. V   AutoGain (1.0 mm/mV)
3: Discrimination AutoGain (1.5 mm/mV)

4: Marqueurs

25 mm/s

❶ Intermittent TWOS is visible following these biventricular paced cycles (Figure 38.2). As the T-waves are not sensed in the far-field discrimination channel (sensing is annotated by VS²), the event is recorded as ventricular oversensing. These cycles are not binned ('–' marker).

❷ Sinus beats detected as ARS events in the PVARP following the oversensed T-waves (note the timing cycles and refractory periods shown at the bottom of the tracing). In this device, AR events are simply indicated by a vertical line, without an 'AR' annotation. ARS events do not reset the AVI timer, leading to loss of biventricular pacing.

Comments

Fortuitus discoveries with a lead noise discrimination algorithm

TWOS was resolved in this case by increasing the duration of the plateau in sensitivity (an alternative would have been to increase the percentage of threshold start)—see Case 28. Inappropriate therapy would not have been delivered as the TWOS cycles were not binned in the VT/VF counters.

Algorithms such as Secure Sense (Abbott) evaluate near-field signals (RV tip to RV ring or RV tip to RV coil) and far-field signals (RV coil to can or RV tip to can) so as to withhold therapy in case of lead integrity issues using a system of counters. The noise counter is incremented with every short cycle in the near-field channel, and reset to 0 following every second (not necessarily consecutive) short cycle on the far-field channel (the cut-off for the short cycles is 400 ms in case of a single VF zone, or the slowest VT cycle + 30 ms). Once the criteria for VT/VF are fulfilled, therapy is withheld if the number of counts on the noise counter is ≥10.

Figure 38.3 Inhibition of inappropriate therapy by the Secure Sense algorithm. The short cycles on the far-field discrimination channel are indicated in blue. When this counter reaches 2, it resets the noise counter in the near-field ventricular channel (shown in red) to 0. Therapy is withheld as the noise counter is ≥10 ('RV lead noise' marker)

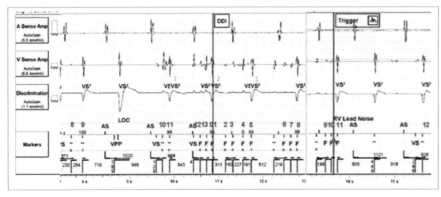

A potential risk of the Secure Sense algorithm is to inappropriately withhold therapy due to undersensing of true ventricular arrhythmia on the discrimination channel. In order to avoid this, the algorithm is automatically reprogrammed to 'Passive' (enabling the delivery of therapy) if one of the three following events occurs in the discrimination channel during an episode: (1) two or more low-amplitude (<0.6 mV) cycles, (2) a pause >2200 ms between two cycles, or (3) occurrence of less than two cycles during the tachycardia.[1]

In addition to its utility to avoid inappropriate shocks due to lead failure, other issues can be diagnosed, such as TWOS (as in the present case), P-wave oversensing, crosstalk, and ventricular non-capture.[2]

References

1. Welte N, Strik M, Eschalier R, et al. Multicenter investigation of an implantable cardioverter-defibrillator algorithm to detect oversensing. *Heart Rhythm* 2017; **14**: 1008–15.
2. Koneru JN, Kaszala K, Bordachar P, Shehata M, Swerdlow C, Ellenbogen KA. Spectrum of issues detected by an ICD diagnostic alert that utilizes far-field electrograms: clinical implications. *Heart Rhythm* 2015; **12**: 957–67.

Introduction to the case

A 53-year-old man attended the emergency department reporting shocks from his ICD followed shortly by syncope. Two weeks prior, he had been implanted with a single-chamber ICD for primary prevention of sudden death in the setting of hypertrophic cardiomyopathy. Past medical history included permanent AF. His device was interrogated in the department and his EGMs are shown in Figure 39.1.

Question

Figure 39.1 Stored arrhythmia episode

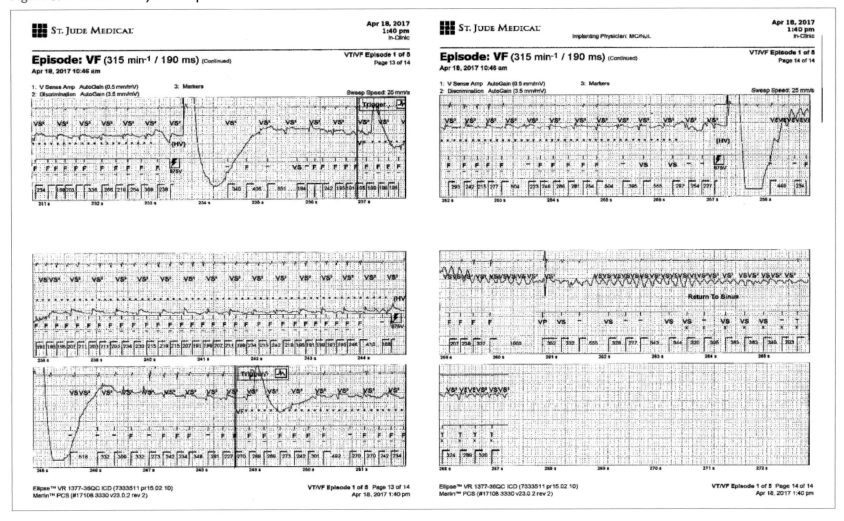

What do you observe?

A Inappropriate shocks due to lead connector issue

B Inappropriate shocks due to lead displacement into the atrium

C Inappropriate shocks due to rapidly conducted AF

D Inappropriate shocks due to TWOS

E Appropriate shocks due to ventricular arrhythmia

Answer

B Inappropriate shocks due to lead displacement into the atrium

Figure 39.2   Annotated tracing

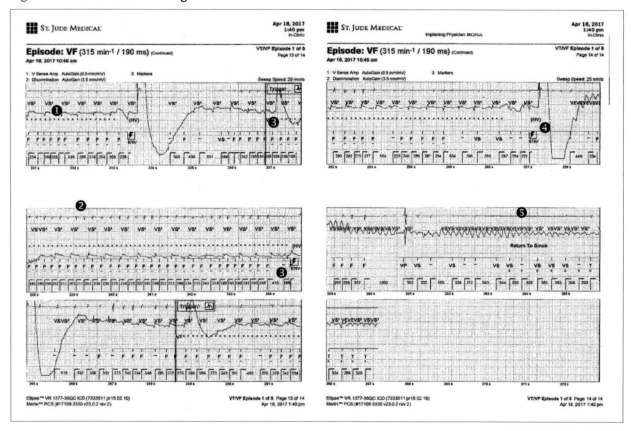

❶ Far-field EGM on the discrimination channel demonstrating irregularly irregular QRS complexes at approximately 150 bpm, representing rapidly conducted AF (Figure 39.2).

❷ Near-field EGM demonstrating discrete, rapid, and irregular activity with cycle lengths between 191 and 220 ms (270–315 bpm). Given that we can see on the far-field EGM that the patient is not in VF, and that the near-field signal is dissociated from the far-field QRS complexes, it has to be sensing AF.

❸ The VS2 markers are part of a mechanism in place to prevent inappropriate therapy in case of sensing issues, but in this instance did not prevent inappropriate shocks due to

low-amplitude signals in the discrimination channel (as a protection against inappropriate inhibition of appropriate therapy due to undersensing in this channel—see Case 38).

❹ Shock on T-wave, inducing VF as seen on the far-field EGM. This is not sensed on the near-field EGM which continues to detect a slower atrial signal.

❺ The AF has been cardioverted, and atrial activity is now sensed below the VT rate, leading the device to interpret a return to normal rhythm despite ongoing VF, visible in the far-field discrimination channel. Further therapy (not shown here) successfully defibrillated the patient.

Comments

Device proarrhythmia

This example illustrates the potentially dramatic consequences of lead dislodgment, and how ICDs may be proarrhythmic.

In addition to inappropriate therapy due to oversensing, other more frequent proarrhythmic effects of ICDs are acceleration of ventricular arrhythmia by ATP or induction of ventricular arrhythmia by inappropriate ATP for supraventricular arrhythmia. ICD shocks in the VT zone are usually delivered as cardioversions (i.e. synchronized to an R-wave) to avoid a T-wave shock with induction of VF. Low-energy (e.g. 5 J) shocks for treatment of VT have also been reported to be proarrhythmic by accelerating the arrhythmia.[1]

Reports of ventricular proarrhythmia induced by implantable devices are due to asynchronous pacing (during magnet application or due to undersensing), short–long–short pacing sequences by ventricular pacing avoidance algorithms,[2] RV pacing in ICD recipients,[3] QT interval prolongation due to LV epicardial pacing,[4] or electrical storm induced by LV pacing adjacent to scar.[5] AF is increased by AAI(R) and VVI(R) pacing compared to DDD(R) pacing,[6,7] and by increased percentages of atrial and ventricular pacing.[8]

Finally, PMT includes:

1 Endless-loop tachycardia.
2 Sensor-driven tachycardia.
3 Tracking of ATs (due to mode switch inactivation, 2:1 locked-in flutter, or intermittent undersensing—see Volume 1, Cases 11 and 25).
4 Atrial oversensing (e.g. of myopotentials) which are tracked, with ventricular pacing.
5 Algorithms such as rate-drop response (see Volume 1, Case 22) and atrial preferential pacing.
6 Runaway PM.

References

1. Sivagangabalan G, Chik W, Zaman S, et al. Antitachycardia pacing for very fast ventricular tachycardia and low-energy shock for ventricular arrhythmias in patients with implantable defibrillators. *Am J Cardiol* 2013; **112**: 1153–7.
2. Sweeney MO, Ruetz LL, Belk P, Mullen TJ, Johnson JW, Sheldon T. Bradycardia pacing-induced short-long-short sequences at the onset of ventricular tachyarrhythmias: a possible mechanism of proarrhythmia? *J Am Coll Cardiol* 2007; **50**: 614–22.
3. Cronin EM, Jones P, Seth MC, Varma N. Right ventricular pacing increases risk of appropriate implantable cardioverter-defibrillator shocks asymmetrically: an analysis of the ALTITUDE database. *Circ Arrhythm Electrophysiol* 2017; **10**: e004711.
4. Bhatia A, Nangia V, Solis J, Dhala A, Sra J, Akhtar M. Biventricular pacing and QT interval prolongation. *J Cardiovasc Electrophysiol* 2007; **18**: 623–7.
5. Roque C, Trevisi N, Silberbauer J, et al. Electrical storm induced by cardiac resynchronization therapy is determined by pacing on epicardial scar and can be successfully managed by catheter ablation. *Circ Arrhythm Electrophysiol* 2014; **7**: 1064–9.
6. Healey JS, Toff WD, Lamas GA, et al. Cardiovascular outcomes with atrial-based pacing compared with ventricular pacing: meta-analysis of randomized trials, using individual patient data. *Circulation* 2006; **114**: 11–17.
7. Nielsen JC, Thomsen PE, Højberg S, et al. A comparison of single-lead atrial pacing with dual-chamber pacing in sick sinus syndrome. *Eur Heart J* 2011; **32**: 686–96.
8. Elkayam LU, Koehler JL, Sheldon TJ, Glotzer TV, Rosenthal LS, Lamas GA. The influence of atrial and ventricular pacing on the incidence of atrial fibrillation: a meta-analysis. *Pacing Clin Electrophysiol* 2011; **34**: 1593–9.

Introduction to the case

A patient with dilated cardiomyopathy and a CRT-D underwent lead revision due to fracture of the ICD lead. A new ICD lead was implanted (see Figure 40.1) and the real-time EGM after lead fixation is shown in Figure 40.2.

Figure 40.1 Peroperative fluoroscopic image in the posteroanterior (PA) and left anterior oblique (LAO) views with position of the new ICD lead (arrows)

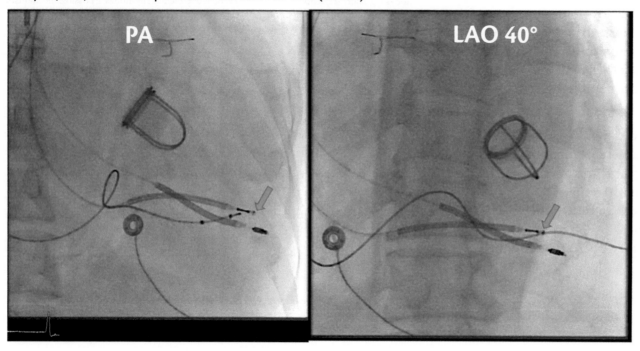

Question

Figure 40.2 Real-time ventricular EGM from the new lead at implantation after the lead was fixated, recorded by the pacing system analyser.

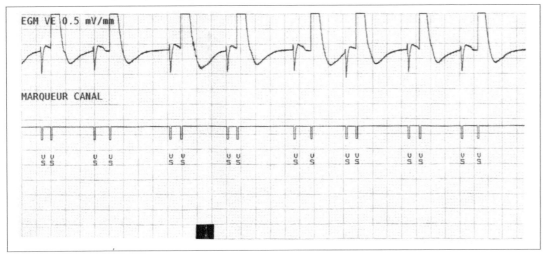

What do you observe?

A Far-field P-wave oversensing

B Lead chatter

C R-wave double counting

D TWOS

E None of the above

Answer

B Lead chatter

Figure 40.3 Annotated tracing

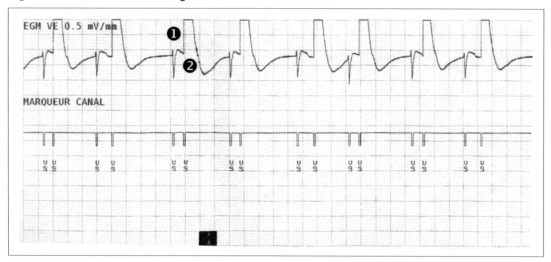

The fluoroscopic image in Figure 40.1 shows integrated bipolar ICD leads (there is no separate ring electrode visible). Although the lead tips are separated, note that the coils cross and are in contact with each other.

❶ The signal in Figure 40.3 corresponds to an artefact resulting from chatter (contact) between the lead coils (the lead tips are at a safe distance from each other and are not responsible for this finding). As these are integrated bipolar leads, the coils are part of the sensing circuit.

❷ The ventricular signal has a current of injury as the lead has just been fixated (the signal is truncated).

Far-field P-waves can sometime be sensed from integrated bipolar leads, but their amplitude would be smaller (measured here at around 5 mV). One would also expect a more constant coupling interval between P- and R-waves. This patient was in permanent AF (note that there is no atrial lead, which would be expected in a patient with CRT in sinus rhythm, and the patient has a Starr mitral valve, indicating long-standing mitral valve disease with a high likelihood of AF).

Comments

Interlead chatter

Chatter between the lead coils was identified in this patient at implantation and repositioning of the new lead solved the issue (Figure 40.4).

Figure 40.4 After repositioning of the new ICD lead (arrows) to avoid contact between the coils (top panels), the artefacts were no longer observed (bottom panel)

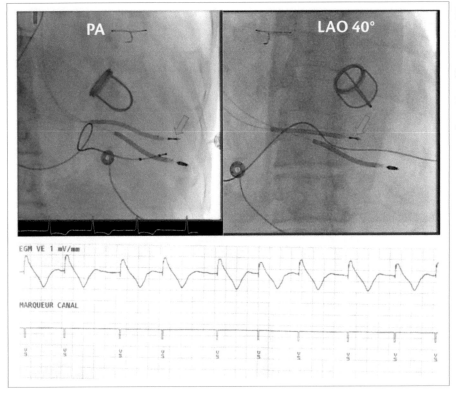

It is important to avoid interlead interaction, which should be evaluated by fluoroscopy and EGM analysis at implantation. Interlead chatter resulting from meta-metal contact can occur between lead tips implanted next to each other, ICD coils,[1] lead fragments,[2] insulation breaches due to erosion between lead bodies,[3] or conductor coil exteriorization.[4]

The consequences of chatter may be inhibition of pacing, inappropriate detection of ventricular arrhythmias, or shunting of current with ineffective shocks.

References

1. Cooper JM, Sauer WH, Garcia FC, Krautkramer MJ, Verdino RJ. Covering sleeves can shield the high-voltage coils from lead chatter in an integrated bipolar ICD lead. *Europace* 2007; **9**: 137–42.
2. Lickfett L, Wolpert C, Jung W, et al. Inappropriate implantable defibrillator discharge caused by a retained pacemaker lead fragment. *J Interv Card Electrophysiol* 1999; **3**: 163–7.
3. Choudhury R, Elsokkari I, Parkash R. Lead-lead interaction: interaction with an abandoned implantable cardiac defibrillator externalized lead. *J Cardiovasc Electrophysiol* 2018; **29**: 1040–1.
4. Kristensen J, Kronborg MB, Lukac P, Nielsen JC. An unusually late dislodged atrial lead catching externalized ICD-lead conductor. A rare cause of simultaneous atrial and ICD lead over-sensing. *J Arrhythm* 2019; **35**: 307–10.

Introduction to the case

A 75-year-old male attends the device clinic having experienced dizziness for a few hours. He had a CRT-D implanted 2 weeks earlier for dilated cardiomyopathy with second-degree AVB. The patient's chest X-ray is shown in Figure 41.1 The EGM from a stored episode is shown in Figure 41.2.

Figure 41.1 Postoperative chest X-ray

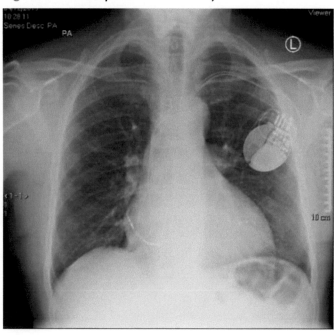

Question

Figure 41.2 Stored arrhythmia episode treated with ATP

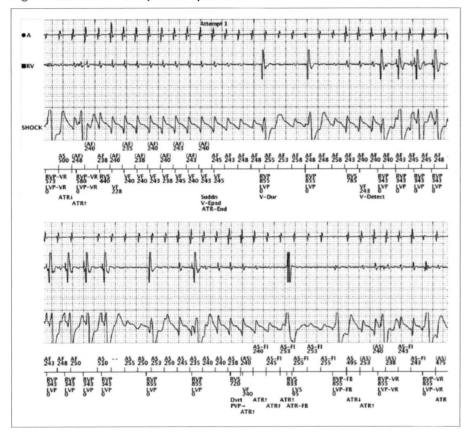

What do you observe?

A AVNRT with inappropriate and unsuccessful ATP

B EMI

C Oversensing of atrial flutter with inappropriate ATP

D RV lead displacement to the atrium

E VT treated by ATP

Answer

C Oversensing of atrial flutter with inappropriate ATP

Figure 41.3 Annotated EGM

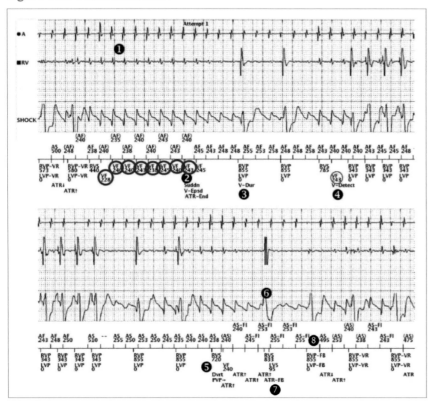

The integrated bipolar ICD lead had been implanted on the interventricular septum, with far-field atrial oversensing of recent-onset atrial flutter.

❶ Near-simultaneous signals on RA and RV EGM with identical cycle length (approximately 240 ms) (Figure 41.3). The signals on the RV EGM correspond to atrial potentials recorded by the integrated bipolar ICD lead straddling the tricuspid annulus. The atrial potentials are sensed in the VF zone and inhibit VP. Note the high-amplitude

ventricular signals on the shock channel, indicating that the lead has not dislodged to the atrium.

❷ In this Boston Scientific ICD, after three fast ventricular events, a sliding detection window opens and evaluates the ten most recent RV RR intervals. Each new interval will be classified as fast (VT or VF) or slow (VP or VS). The 'VEpsd' marker appears after 8/10 fast events (blue circles) with fulfilment of the onset criterion ('Suddn' marker), which is more than the programmed threshold of 9%. This marker also starts the duration timer, which increments as long as 6/10 fast intervals are detected.

❸ The 'VDur' marker indicates (1) the end of the duration timer (nominally set to 1 s in the VF zone in this device), (2) the detection window has remained satisfied by ≥6/10 fast intervals, and (3) detection of an arrhythmic episode has not yet been satisfied (otherwise, a 'V-Detect' marker would have been shown). The reason for this is that biventricular pacing was delivered after a period without atrial oversensing (i.e. there was a 'slow' event). Reasons that 'Vdur' appears instead of 'V-Detect' are:

- the last beat of the duration timer is slow (i.e. VP or VS)
- the last beat of the duration timer does not match the zone where 8/10 was met
- detection enhancements determine that this is SVT (however, in the VF zone in this device, no detection enhancements are applied)
- the rhythm fell in the 'Monitor Only zone'
- a magnet is on the device.

❹ The 'V-detect' marker indicates that (1) duration has timed out and (2) the detection window as remained satisfied by ≥6/10 fast intervals—in this case, 7/10 intervals are fast. In the VF zone, the 'last in zone' criterion should also be met with the last beat in the detection window being fast, which is the case with the VF event (red circle). Burst ATP is delivered before charging.

❺ The device checks whether ≥2/3 fast events are present after ATP. As this is not the case, therapy is diverted ('Dvrt' marker) and the capacitors are not charged. Diverted therapy is accompanied by PVARP extension to 400 ms for one cycle ('PVP→' marker).

❻ Intrinsic ventricular activity is sensed in both ventricular channels.

❼ Due to the high atrial rate, the device mode switches to a VDIR mode ('ATR-FB' marker).

❽ Biventricular pacing in VDIR mode at the programmed lower rate of 70 bpm during modeswitch.

Comments

Atrial oversensing with integrated bipolar implantable cardioverter defibrillator leads

As the RV coil is part of the sensing circuit in integrated bipolar ICD leads (there is no ring electrode, as opposed to true/dedicated bipolar ICD leads), these leads are prone to atrial oversensing if the coil straddles the tricuspid annulus.

Ablating the flutter would not solve the issue, as atrial oversensing is likely to persist in sinus rhythm or in AF.

Therapeutic options to prevent oversensing with inhibition of pacing and inappropriate ICD therapy in this case would include: (1) reducing ventricular sensitivity (however, with a risk of ventricular undersensing), (2) exchanging the lead for a true bipolar model (however, it is in general recommended to match the manufacturer of the ICD generator with that of the lead to avoid technical issues[1]) or (3) repositioning the lead (e.g. at the apex). The last option is probably the best and should be feasible as the lead had been implanted recently and may be easily mobilized.

Integrated bipolar leads (only manufactured by Boston Scientific) are robust and have been shown to reduce TWOS.[2] This sensing configuration can also be programmed in dedicated bipolar leads in some device models (e.g. Medtronic) to troubleshoot TWOS or in case of low sensing amplitude with true bipolar sensing. However, integrated bipolar leads may be complicated by P-wave oversensing in as much as 11% of cases,[3] and signal quality should be carefully evaluated at implantation, especially if the lead is positioned on the interventricular septum (as in the present case), in which instance the coil may straddle the tricuspid annulus. Furthermore, integrated bipolar sensing with leads implanted at the apex may be prone to diaphragmatic myopotential oversensing (see Volume 1, Case 45).[4]

References

1. Burri H, Starck C, Auricchio A, et al. EHRA expert consensus statement and practical guide on optimal implantation technique for conventional pacemakers and implantable cardioverter defibrillators. *Europace* 2021; **23**: 983–1008.
2. Rodríguez-Mañero M, de Asmundis C, Sacher F, et al. T-wave oversensing in patients with Brugada syndrome: true bipolar versus integrated bipolar implantable cardioverter defibrillator leads: multicenter retrospective study. *Circ Arrhythm Electrophysiol* 2015; **8**: 792–8.
3. Weretka S, Michaelsen J, Becker R, et al. Ventricular oversensing: a study of 101 patients implanted with dual chamber defibrillators and two different lead systems. *Pacing Clin Electrophysiol* 2003; **26**: 65–70.
4. Schulte B, Sperzel J, Carlsson J, et al. Inappropriate arrhythmia detection in implantable defibrillator therapy due to oversensing of diaphragmatic myopotentials. *J Interv Card Electrophysiol* 2001; **5**: 487–93.

Introduction to the case

A 68-year-old man attends the pacing clinic following an unprovoked syncopal episode. He had a VVI ICD implanted 4 years previously for ischaemic cardiomyopathy (NYHA class II) with severe LV systolic dysfunction and normal QRS duration. His device settings and rate histogram are shown in Figure 42.1, and the EGM of a retrieved episode is shown in Figure 42.2.

Figure 42.1 Device settings and rate histogram

VT/VF Detection

		V. Interval (Rate)	Initial	Redetect
VF	On	270 ms (222 bpm)	30/40	12/16
FVT	OFF			
VT	OFF	360 ms (167 bpm)	16	12
Monitor	Monitor	360 ms (167 bpm)	32	

Wavelet		**Other Enhancements**	
Wavelet	On	Stability	Off
Template	17-Nov-2017	Onset	Off
Match Threshold	70 %	High Rate Timeout	
Auto Collection	On	VF Zone Only	Off
SVT V Limit	260 ms	TWave	On
		RV Lead Noise	On+Timeout
		Timeout	0.75 min

Pacing Summary

Mode		**Rates**	
Mode	VVI	Lower	40 bpm

Pacing Details	**RV**
Amplitude	2.75 V
Pulse Width	0.40 ms
Capture Management	Adaptive
Amplitude Margin	2.0 X
Min. Adapted Amplitude	2.00 V
Acute Phase Remaining	Off
Acute Phase Completed	17-Nov-2017
Sensitivity	0.30 mV
Pace Polarity	Bipolar
Sense Polarity	Bipolar

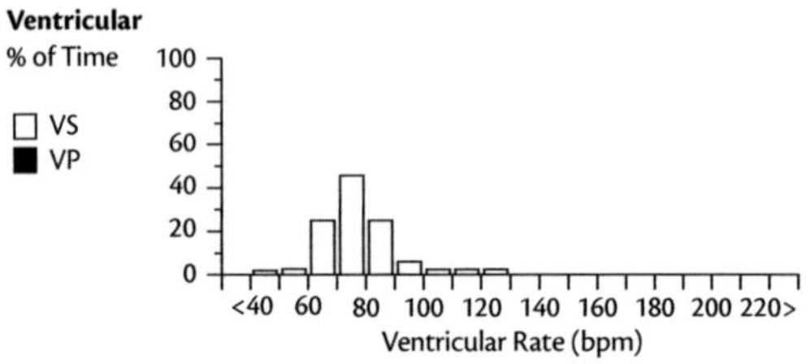
Ventricular
% of Time
VS
VP
100
80
60
40
20
0
<40 60 80 100 120 140 160 180 200 220>
Ventricular Rate (bpm)

Question

Figure 42.2 EGM of retrieved episode

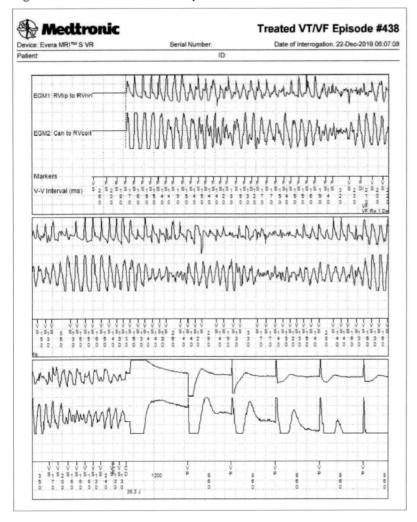

What changes should be made in view of ventricular pacing?

A Enable hysteresis rate

B No change

C Reduce beta-blocker dose

D Turn on rate response

E Upgrade to CRT-D

Answer

B No change

Figure 42.3   Annotated EGM

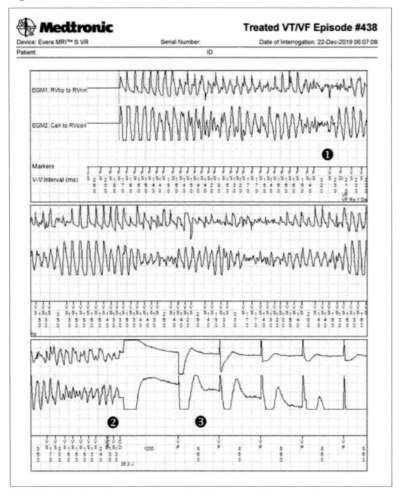

❶ Both the near-field and far-field EGMS demonstrate rapid, coarse electrical activity with variable cycle length (Figure 42.3), in keeping with VF. Note the VS event before fibrillation detection ('FD') due to transient undersensing of low-amplitude potentials. This device utilizes a 'probabilistic counter' in the VF zone whereby only 30/40 beats need to be within the VF zone for the device to detect tachycardia (although the programmed rate of 222 bpm is higher than the tested and currently recommended limit of 188–200 bpm[1]). Had this been a 'consecutive counter' as seen in VT zones for this particular device, the counter would have reset and detection would have been delayed. All devices utilize some form of probabilistic counter or rolling average in the VF zone, so that detection is not delayed in the event of transient undersensing due to variable signal amplitude of fibrillation waves. The benefit of a consecutive counter is that it may reduce inappropriate therapy for rapidly conducted AF whereby one longer RR interval below the tachycardia zone would reset the counter.

❷ Delivery of a non-committed 36.3 J shock for VF, successfully terminating the arrhythmia.

❸ VP at 70 bpm (860 ms). Note the programmed base rate of 40 bpm. This is due to post-shock pacing. This is programmable and is typically at a relatively brisk rate with high output to ensure electrical capture (in this device programmed 6 V at 1.5 ms).

Comments

Post-shock pacing

The patient did not have a pacing indication previously and we can see from his heart rate histograms that he is never paced with the current settings (i.e. rate hysteresis is unnecessary). Therefore, rate response does not need to be activated. Reducing his beta-blocker dose would not prevent post-shock pacing and would be potentially deleterious given the underlying ischaemic cardiomyopathy.

Post-shock pacing is a programmable option whereby the device temporarily delivers VP at a relatively brisk rate following defibrillation for VT/VF to increase cardiac output following the no/low-flow during arrhythmia. This is typically at high pacing voltage and broad pulse width to ensure capture. The benefit of post-shock pacing remains unproven, with the majority of patients not requiring pacing following defibrillation. There are, however, rare cases of defibrillation resulting in bradyarrhythmia which may contribute towards death following successful defibrillation.

Reference

1. Stiles MK, Fauchier L, Morillo CA, Wilkoff BL. 2019 HRS/EHRA/APHRS/LAHRS focused update to 2015 expert consensus statement on optimal implantable cardioverter-defibrillator programming and testing. *Europace* 2019; **21**: 1442–3.

Introduction to the case

A patient with dilated cardiomyopathy was implanted with a dual-chamber
ICD for primary prevention of sudden death. The patient was asymptomatic.
An arrythmia episode was retrieved from the device memory. The tachogram
is shown in Figure 43.1 and the EGM in Figure 43.2.

Figure 43.1 Tachogram of the arrhythmic episode retrieved at device interrogation

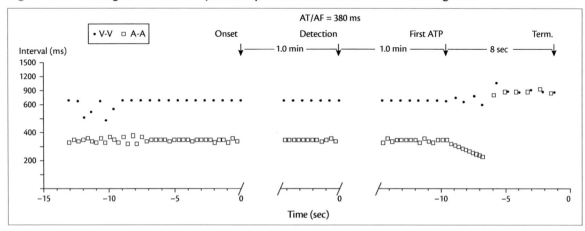

Question

Figure 43.2 EGM retrieved by device interrogation

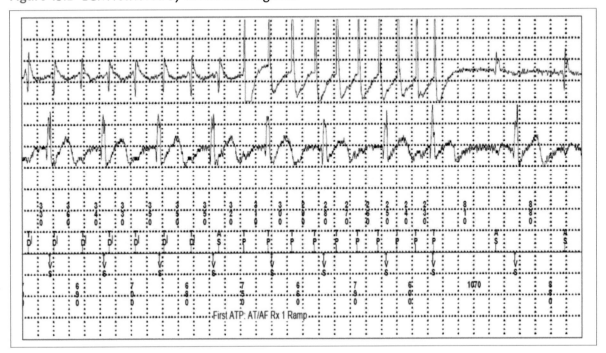

Which statement is true?

A Algorithm only available in ICDs

B AT/atrial flutter terminated by ramp ATP

C AVNRT terminated by ATP

D AVRT terminated by ramp ATP

E Dual tachycardia terminated by ATP

Answer

B AT/atrial flutter terminated by ramp ATP

Figure 43.3 Annotated tracing

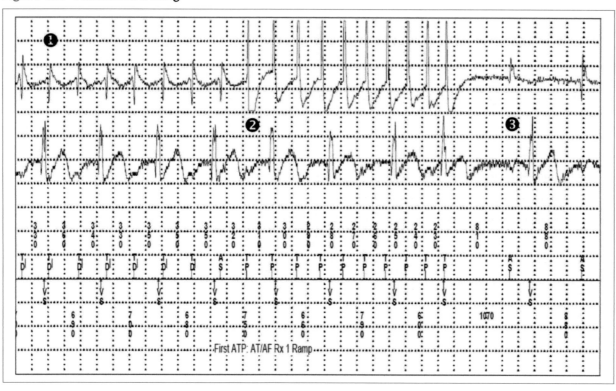

AT/atrial flutter with 2:1 conduction is successfully treated with atrial ramp ATP. This feature is available in certain PMs and ICDs.

❶ AT/ atrial flutter with 2:1 conduction (Figure 43.3). AVNRT with 2:1 response is possible but is a rare finding, and VA intervals would be expected to be more constant. A 1:1 AV ratio is obligatory with AVRT.

❷ Atrial ramp ATP is delivered after fulfilment of the tachycardia detection criteria.

❸ Return to sinus rhythm.

Comments

Atrial antitachycardia pacing algorithms

A number of algorithms are available to prevent atrial arrhythmias (e.g. continuous atrial overdrive pacing) which have been shown to have a slight[1,2] or no[3] effect on atrial arrhythmias. Some pacemaker and ICDs also have atrial overdrive pacing algorithms (burst and/or ramp) to treat atrial arrhythmias, which can sometimes be effective for treating AT or atrial flutter. These algorithms should only be activated at follow-up once the lead has stabilized, to avoid rapid ventricular pacing in case of lead dislodgment (the algorithm will be activated by erroneous detection of atrial tachyarrhythmia due to dislodgement near the tricuspid annulus with A+V sensing, or due to TWOS). Devices nevertheless have safety features such as an atrial lead position check test (with diagnosis of atrial lead dislodgment based upon very short AP–VS delays) and may also inactivate therapies if atrial ATP increases the ventricular rate.

Manual delivery of bursts may also be performed with non-invasive pacing studies to confirm right- or left-sided flutter (with a post-pacing interval minus tachycardia cycle length >100 ms in case of left-sided atrial flutter[4]) or for overdriving the arrhythmia during an in-office visit.

References

1. Carlson MD, Ip J, Messenger J, Beau S, et al. A new pacemaker algorithm for the treatment of atrial fibrillation: results of the Atrial Dynamic Overdrive Pacing Trial (ADOPT). *Journal of the American College of Cardiology* 2003; **42**: 627–33.
2. Boriani G, Tukkie R, Manolis AS, et al. Atrial antitachycardia pacing and managed ventricular pacing in bradycardia patients with paroxysmal or persistent atrial tachyarrhythmias: the MINERVA randomized multicentre international trial. *Eur Heart J* 2014; **35**: 2352–62.
3. Healey JS, Connolly SJ, Gold MR, et al. Subclinical atrial fibrillation and the risk of stroke. *N Engl J Med* 2012; **366**: 120–9.
4. Burri H, Zimmermann M, Sunthorn H, et al. Noninvasive pacing study via pacemakers and implantable cardioverter-defibrillators for differentiating right from left atrial flutter. *Heart Rhythm* 2015; **12**: 1221–6.

Introduction to the case

An 18-year-old youth, implanted with a subcutaneous implantable cardioverter defibrillator (S-ICD) for idiopathic VF, consulted after having received a shock preceded by palpitations. A stored event was retrieved from the device memory. The tracing of the event is shown in Figure 44.1. Device settings are presented in Table 44.1.

Table 44.1 Device settings

Therapy	On
Shock zone	250 bpm
Conditional shock zone	190 bpm
Post-shock pacing	On
SMART Pass	On
Gain setting	1×
Sensing configuration	Primary
Shock polarity	STD

Question

Figure 44.1 Tracing of the treated event

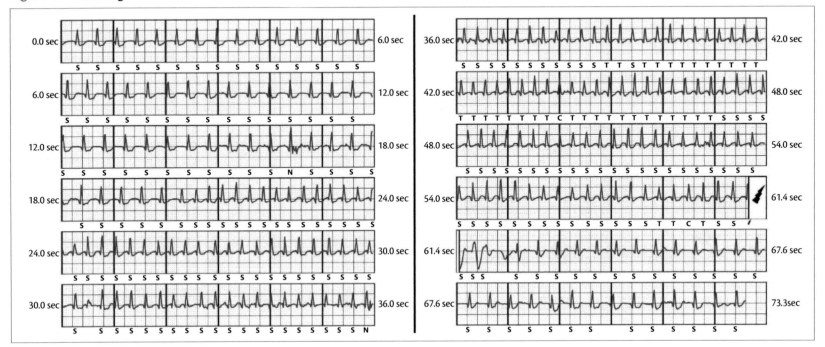

What programming changes would you recommend?

A Activate AF discrimination algorithm

B Decrease conditional zone to 180 bpm

C Increase conditional zone to 220 bpm

D Programme a different sensing vector

E None of the above

Answer

E None of the above

Figure 44.2 Annotated tracing

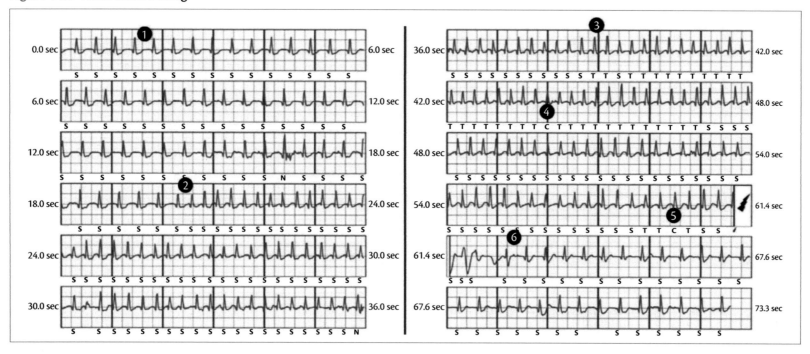

❶ The subcutaneous electrocardiogram (S-ECG) (Figure 44.2) shows a regular rhythm with ventricular events labelled as 'S'. The underlying rhythm is probably sinus tachycardia at approximately 150–160 bpm. The calculated heart rate is below the programmed conditional zone rate cut-off, the detection marker is 'S'.

❷ A sudden increase in rate can be observed; rate is approximately 215 bpm which is detected in the conditional zone. During this fast rhythm, the ventricular events are appropriately labelled as 'S' because of the morphology or width criteria. Therefore, changing the sensing vector is not necessary.

❸ The cycles are automatically labelled as 'T' because the calculated average cycle rate is above the programmed shock zone rate cut-off (which is already set to the maximum programmable value of 250 bpm).

❹ Detection criteria are fulfilled and the device starts charging (first 'C' marker).

❺ The second 'C' marker indicates that at the end of the charge cycle, the shock confirmation algorithm is satisfied and the device tops off the capacitor charge to deliver a synchronized committed shock.

❻ After the shock, the rhythm is restored to sinus tachycardia (after two ventricular beats).

Comments

Subcutaneous implantable cardioverter defibrillator inappropriate shocks due to supraventricular tachycardia

The S-ICD algorithm architecture consists of three phases:

1 The detection phase filters subcutaneous electrocardiogram (S-ECG) signals and detections are identified (no markers are generated during this phase).
2 The certification phase determines if the waveforms associated with the declared events are cardiac in nature (waveform appraisal). During the certification phase, four double detection algorithms are employed to discard over-sensed detections (i.e. TWOS) and certified heart rate is determined.
3 The decision phase performs rate evaluation and rhythm discrimination using static and dynamic correlation waveform analysis. First, the cycle rate is calculated using a running average of the four previous intervals denoted by certified detections. Every certified detection is annotated as an 'S' (sensed or sinus) or a 'T' (treatable) detection, depending on the cycle rate and zone programming. If the rate is in the conditional zone, additional morphology match and QRS width criteria are applied. If the rate is in the shock zone, the rhythm will automatically be 'T' (treatable).

There are no specific S-ICD discrimination algorithms for rapidly conducted supraventricular arrhythmias. In the present case, the issue was that rapid cycles were automatically classified as 'T' due to their rate falling in the shock zone. Therefore, management of the supraventricular arrhythmia, either with curative ablation or with drugs (antiarrhythmic or rate slowing) would be the best course of action in this patient. Recurrence of AF may be detected by an algorithm which monitors RR irregularity, but it is important to note that S-ICDs currently do not have monitoring zones, and only non-sustained tachycardia episodes which elicit a first 'C' marker are stored in the device memory.

Introduction to the case

A 29-year-old man, implanted with an S-ICD for secondary prevention of sudden death, presented for routine follow-up with several bouts of dizziness and palpitations. Device settings are shown in Table 45.1. An arrhythmic episode was retrieved from the device memory and the S-ECG is shown in Figure 45.1.

Table 45.1 Device settings

Therapy	On
Shock zone	220 bpm
Conditional shock zone	190 bpm
Post-shock pacing	On
SMART Charge	2.88 s (11 intervals)
Gain setting	1×
Sensing configuration	Primary
Shock polarity	STD

Question

Figure 45.1 S-ECG of the retrieved event

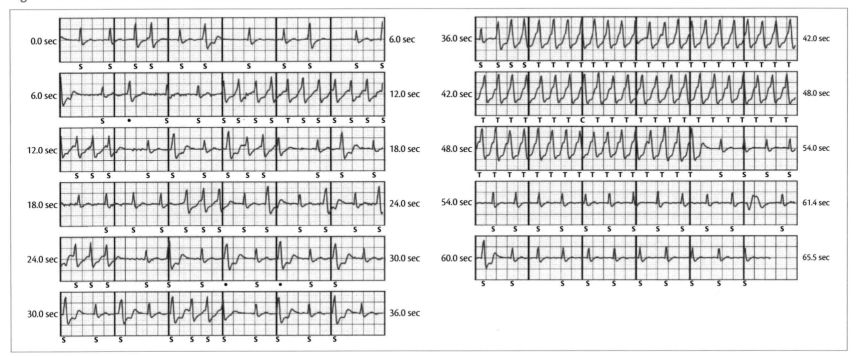

What is your diagnosis?

A Appropriately aborted shock

B Appropriately delivered shock

C Dropped charge due to exceeded charge time

D Inappropriately aborted shock

E Inappropriately delivered shock

Answer

A Appropriately aborted shock

Figure 45.2 Annotated S-ECG

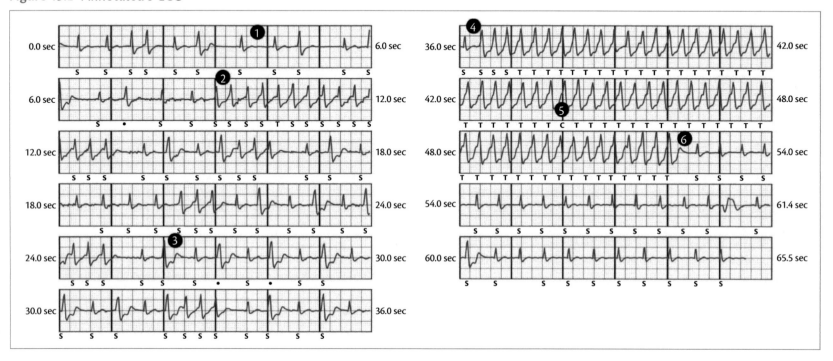

❶ The S-ECG (Figure 45.2) shows a rhythm with narrow and wide ventricular events labelled as 'S' or '•'. The underlying rhythm is sinus tachycardia at approximately 100 bpm with ventricular premature beats.

❷ At timestamps 9–13 s, a non-sustained VT of 14 complexes occurs. The running average of four detected events is below the lowest programmed rate cut-off, except for one ventricular event labelled as 'T', the others are labelled 'S'.

❸ Sinus rhythm with ventricular bigeminy is observed.

❹ VT occurs. The fourth detected event is labelled as 'T' as the running average of detected events is above the programmed rate cut-off of the shock zone.

❺ After detection is fulfilled, the device starts charging the capacitors ('C' marker).

❻ Spontaneous termination of the VT after 8 s of charging. As the shock confirmation algorithm is not fulfilled, the charge is aborted (there is no marker to indicate when this occurs). Due to spontaneous termination of the tachyarrhythmia, SMART Charge will be applied for the next detected event. SMART Charge will extend the detection time/number of detected beats for initial detection, in order to prevent charging of the capacitors for non-sustained arrhythmias.

Comments

Non-sustained ventricular arrhythmias with subcutaneous implantable cardioverter defibrillators

Non-sustained episodes which elicit a capacitor charge with an aborted shock will extend the number of beats required for detection after the 18/24 counter is fulfilled, from 2 to up to 17 beats in increments of 3 beats ('Smart Charge' feature). This patient has had three previous non-sustained episodes which elicited a capacitor charge, as indicated by Smart Charge (extension of 11 intervals).

It is important to note that current generations of S-ICDs do not have monitor-only VT zones. Ventricular arrhythmias, sustained or non-sustained, will only be stored if a capacitor charge is initiated. Smart Pass episodes (i.e. identification of TWOS) or AF episodes will, however, store S-ECGs.

Introduction to the case

A 30-year-old man with a hypertrophic cardiomyopathy and a history of non-sustained VT had been implanted with an S-ICD for primary prevention of sudden death. He consulted after having received a shock. A stored event was retrieved from the device memory. Programmed parameters are shown in Table 46.1 and the S-ECG of the event is displayed in Figure 46.1.

Table 46.1 Device settings

Therapy	On
Shock zone	230 bpm
Conditional shock zone	180 bpm
Post-shock pacing	On
SMART Pass	Off
Gain setting	1×
Sensing configuration	Alternate
Shock polarity	STD

Question

Figure 46.1 S-ECG of the treated event

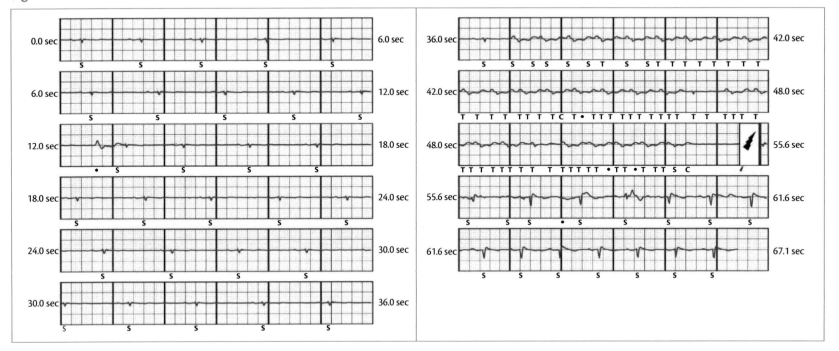

What is your diagnosis?

A Appropriate shock for VF

B Appropriate shock for fast VT

C Inappropriate shock for AF

D Inappropriate shock for cardiac oversensing

E Inappropriate shock for non-cardiac oversensing

Answer

D Inappropriate shock for cardiac oversensing

Figure 46.2 Annotated tracing

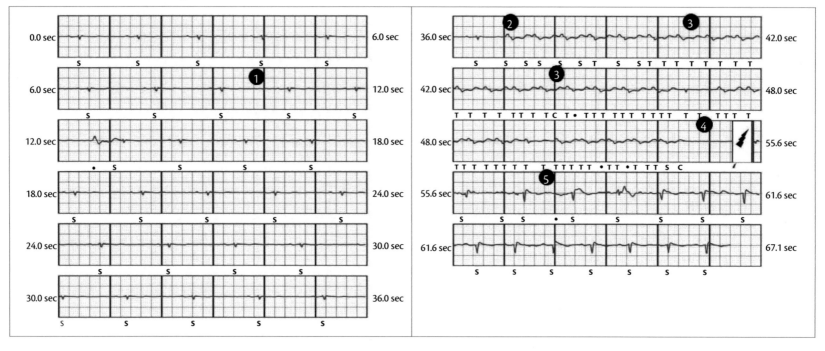

❶ The S-ECG (Figure 46.2) shows ventricular events labelled as 'S', which are detected cardiac events. The underlying rhythm is sinus bradycardia at approximately 45–50 bpm.

❷ A stable slow VT at rate of 120 bpm is initiated. Both the QRS complex and intermittently the T-wave are detected and are labelled 'S' as the running average of four detections is below the programmed conditional zone rate cut-off.

❸ From timestamp 39 s onwards, cardiac oversensing (TWOS and R-wave double counting) is more prevalent. The detected events are labelled 'T' because the calculated average rate is above the programmed shock zone rate cut-off. At timestamp 44 s, detection is fulfilled and the device starts charging (first 'C' marker).

❹ Charging is completed (not indicated by a marker) and the 'shock confirmation' algorithm is satisfied at 52.4 s (second 'C' marker). Thereafter, a short charge cycle 'tops off' the capacitors, and an 80 J shock is delivered, which is inappropriate (although it may be argued that this was truly VT).

❺ Post shock, the S-ECG shows sinus rhythm at 75–80 bpm.

Comments

Troubleshooting subcutaneous implantable cardioverter defibrillator
T-wave oversensing

TWOS is one of the most common causes for inappropriate S-ICD shocks. The issue has been partially addressed with the advent of the SMART Pass algorithm.[1] This is a 9 Hz high-pass filter which attenuates low-frequency signals such as the T-wave. However, as this filter also reduces QRS amplitude, it is automatically inactivated when the device detects R-waves which are of low amplitude (five consecutive cycles of <0.25 mV with at least two RR intervals of >1.4 s). It is also automatically inactivated if asystole of at least 10 s is detected. During sensing vector selection, SMART Pass will be activated if the chosen vector has R-wave amplitudes ≥0.5 mV. Currently, SMART Pass needs to be manually reactivated in these situations.

Another aspect is that signal detection has different properties depending on the detection zone. In the shock zone (where most instances of TWOS fall), sensing is the most aggressive, in order to detect low-amplitude, fast rhythms. This factor may further enhance propensity to TWOS.

This patient had low-amplitude QRS complexes, which explains the automatic inactivation of SMART Pass. The slow VT was also of low amplitude, which, combined with inactivation of SMART Pass, predisposed to TWOS. It would be advisable to perform a vector check to evaluate whether an alternative vector would yield better sensing.

As QRS and T-wave amplitude may change with exercise, some physicians perform a stress test to evaluate whether this is an issue at higher heart rates in selected patients (routine stress testing has, however, not been shown to be useful[2]). Ideally, a heart rate of at least 168 bpm should be reached, as sensing becomes more aggressive at this rate (and yet more aggressive as from the programmed conditional zone), which may predispose to TWOS. Nominal sensitivity only reverts once the heart rate falls below 150 bpm (sensing hysteresis). If TWOS is detected during exercise and cannot be solved by changing sensing vectors, a template may be taken manually during tachycardia.

References

1. Theuns DAMJ, Brouwer TF, Jonse PW, et al. Prospective blinded evaluation of a novel sensing methodology designed to reduce inappropriate shocks by the subcutaneous implantable cardioverter-defibrillator. *Heart Rhythm* 2018;**15**:1515–22.
2. Afzal MR, Evenson C, Badin A, et al. Role of exercise electrocardiogram to screen for T-wave oversensing after implantation of subcutaneous implantable cardioverter-defibrillator. *Heart Rhythm* 2017; **14**: 1436–9.

Introduction to the case

A 35-year-old woman implanted 2 years ago with an S-ICD for syncopal sustained polymorphic VT presented with a shock while practising yoga. Device parameters are shown in Figure 47.1. Her tracing retrieved from the device memory is shown in Figure 47.2.

Figure 47.1 Current device parameters

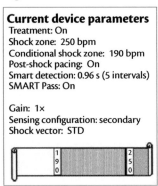

Current device parameters
Treatment: On
Shock zone: 250 bpm
Conditional shock zone: 190 bpm
Post-shock pacing: On
Smart detection: 0.96 s (5 intervals)
SMART Pass: On

Gain: 1×
Sensing configuration: secondary
Shock vector: STD

Question

Figure 47.2 Tracing of arrhythmic episode retrieved from the device memory

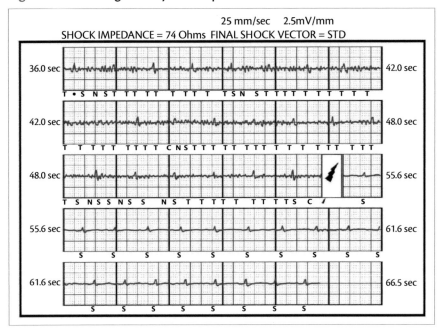

What is the most likely explanation for the shock?

A Circuitry problem

B EMI

C Lead fracture

D Lead connection issue

E Myopotentials

Answer

E Myopotentials

Figure 47.3 Annotated tracing

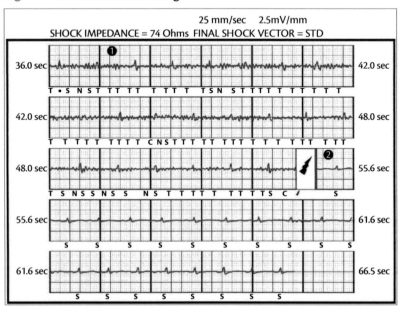

❶ Low-amplitude, high-frequency signals are visible (Figure 47.3) and correspond to myopotentials (the patient was in a position with isometric contraction of the torso). The signals are sensed intermittently and detected as tachycardia cycles (T) or noise (N). Myopotential oversensing is favoured by the relatively low-amplitude QRS complexes.

❷ A shock is delivered upon which the patient immediately relaxes, with disappearance of the myopotentials. Lead fracture or EMI would have persisted after the shock.

Regarding the device parameters shown in Figure 47.1, in case of very low QRS amplitude or long intervals, the Smart Pass algorithm (designed to avoid TWOS) is automatically disabled, which was not the case here. 'Smart Charge' had extended detection from the initial value of two intervals up to five intervals, which implies that a charge cycle occurred, but the shock was not delivered, due to non-sustained events (either non-sustained arrhythmias or intermittent myopotential oversensing).

Comments

Myopotential oversensing with S-ICDs

As S-ICDs analyse surface ECG signals, they are prone to myopotential oversensing, which is nevertheless rare due to filters and device recognition of noise. The generator (usually implanted in an intermuscular pocket) is an integral part of the sensing circuit in the primary and secondary vectors. Therefore, these two vectors are more prone to this issue. As is often the case, the alternate vector in this patient yielded QRS signals which were of very low amplitude (Figure 47.4). Low signal amplitude will also predispose to myopotential oversensing, and it is important to verify proper sensing with different postures during the automatic setup. When R-wave amplitudes are consistently low, one can consider using the gain setting 2× which can increase the likelihood that the device will classify the myopotentials as 'N' (noise). In this patient, 2× gain resulted in a risk of signal clipping, which did not allow this setting.

Figure 47.4 Sensing vectors of S-ICDs with corresponding signals in the present case

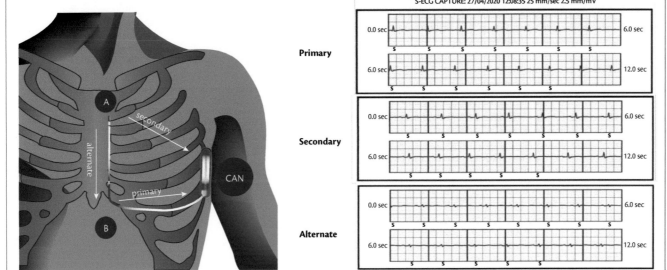

Even though the alternate vector does not involve the generator, signals from this vector may also have myopotential oversensing issues if the lead is not medial enough and overlies the pectoral muscle.

In this patient, the amplitude of myopotentials upon isometric contraction of the torso was similar in the primary and secondary configurations, and it was decided to keep the sensing vector in the secondary configuration. The patient was advised to avoid exercises with prolonged contraction of the torso muscles.

Introduction to the case

A patient with a S-ICD received a shock while driving his car. He had no complaints preceding the shock. The tracings retrieved from the device memory are shown in Figure 48.1.

Question

Figure 48.1 Episode retrieved from the S-ICD

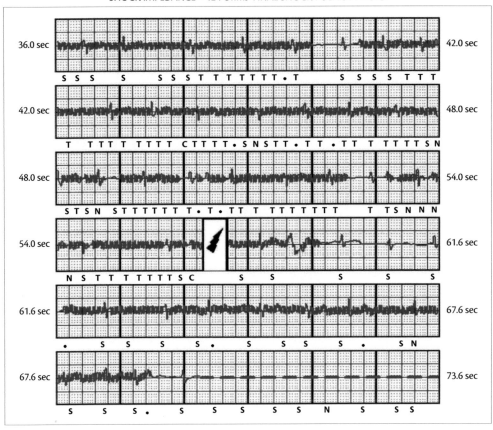

SHOCK IMPEDANCE = 124 Ohms FINAL SHOCK POLARITY = STD

What is the most appropriate action?

A Activate SMART Pass filter

B Change sensing vector

C Eliminate source of EMI

D Implant a transvenous ICD

E Reposition the lead

Answer

C Eliminate source of EMI

Figure 48.2 Annotated tracing

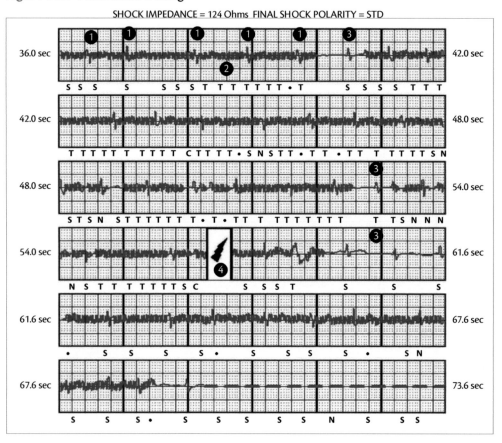

The tracing in Figure 48.2 shows high-frequency signals suggestive of EMI which was caused by a malfunctioning car seat heating system, and which led to inappropriate shock.

❶ QRS complexes are visible, with superimposed EMI.

❷ Oversensing of the EMI ('T' markers).

❸ Short pauses in the noise revealing normal detection of QRS.

❹ A shock is delivered without change in the noise.

Comments

Oversensing by S-ICDs

In transvenous ICD systems, the main reason for inappropriate therapy is rapidly conducted SVT (especially AF), and to a lesser extent, R-wave oversensing or TWOS and EMI. In the S-ICD system, oversensing is the most important reason for inappropriate therapy, whereas SVTs only play a minor role.[1,2,3] The different reasons for oversensing include myopotentials, EMI, and TWOS. Low QRS amplitude favours oversensing due to automatic gain settings.

The S-ICD system may be prone to myopotential oversensing because the sensing electrodes and generator (part of the primary and secondary sensing vectors) are implanted close to skeletal muscles. Myopotential oversensing is possible with any of the vectors, depending on the type of exercise being performed.[4]

Oversensing of EMI may be favoured by the large sensing bipole.

TWOS has been reduced by the advent of the SMART Pass filter, which, however, is not designed to eliminate occurrence of myopotential or EMI oversensing.

References

1. Olde Nordkamp LR, Brouwer TF, Barr C, et al. Inappropriate shocks in the subcutaneous ICD: incidence, predictors and management. *Int J Cardiol* 2015; **195**: 126–33.
2. Rudic B, Tülümen E, Fastenrath F, et al. Incidence, mechanisms, and clinical impact of inappropriate shocks in patients with a subcutaneous defibrillator. *Europace* 2020; **22**: 761–8.
3. Theuns DAM, Brouwer TF, Jones P, et al. A prospective, blinded evaluation of a novel sensing methodology designed to reduce inappropriate shocks by the subcutaneous implantable defibrillator. *Heart Rhythm* 2018; 15: 1515–22.
4. van den Bruck JH, Sultan A, Plenge T, et al. Incidence of myopotential induction in subcutaneous implantable cardioverter-defibrillator patients: is the oversensing issue really solved? *Heart Rhythm* 2019; 16: 1523–30.

Introduction to the case

A 50-year-old man was scheduled for implantation of a S-ICD for secondary prevention of sudden death. After implantation, he experienced a shock without preceding symptoms at the ward. The stored event was retrieved from the device memory and is shown in Figure 49.1. The device settings are presented in Table 49.1.

Table 49.1 Device settings

Therapy	ON
Shock zone	250 bpm
Conditional shock zone	180 bpm
Post shock pacing	ON
SMART Pass	OFF
Gain setting	1 X
Sensing configuration	Primary
Shock polarity	STD

Question

Figure 49.1 Stored event

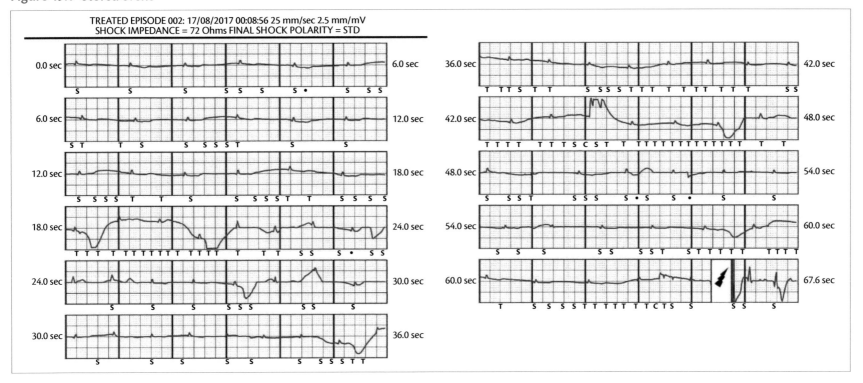

What is your diagnosis?

A Air entrapment

B EMI

C Lead fracture

D Loose set-screw

E Myopotentials

Answer

A Air entrapment

Figure 49.2 Annotated tracing

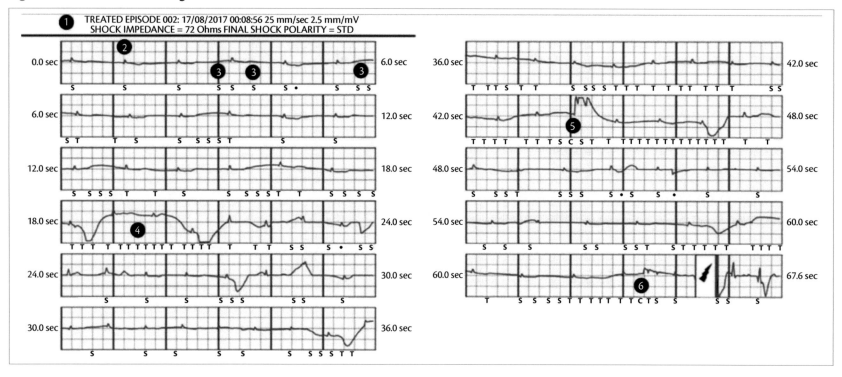

The patient experienced inappropriate shock shortly after implantation due to artefacts resulting from air entrapment, which resulted in the characteristic wandering of the baseline (Figure 49.2).

❶ The episode text contains information on the event, included the measured shock impedance of 72 ohms, which is normal and points against lead fracture (which would be unusual so soon after implantation) or a loose set-screw.

❷ The tracing shows ventricular events labelled as 'S', which are detected cardiac events. The underlying rhythm is sinus rhythm at approximately 60 bpm.

❸ Some events labelled as 'S' are unrelated to QRS complexes. The heart rate is determined by the running average of four detected events. When the rate is above the shock zone or above the conditional shock zone with poor morphology/width match according to the discriminators, detected events are indicated 'T', otherwise they are indicated 'S'. Of note, baseline wander of the S-ECG is present which becomes more marked.

❹ More events are labelled as 'T' due to extreme baseline wander of the S-ECG.

❺ Detection is fulfilled and a charge marker 'C' is visible at 44 s. The device starts charging the capacitor.

❻ The second 'C' marker at 63.4 s indicates that at the end of the charge cycle, the shock confirmation algorithm is satisfied, and the device tops off the capacitor charge to deliver a synchronized committed shock.

Comments

Inappropriate subcutaneous implantable cardioverter defibrillator shock due to air entrapment

Inappropriate shocks may occur early after implantation and highlight the importance of good tissue contact of the electrodes to prevent inappropriate shocks. The presence of air in the pocket or the lead tunnel insulates the sensing contact ring, causing inadequate sensing and low-amplitude signals, and thus oversensing from autogain. Care must be taken during implantation to avoid residual air pockets by flushing with saline and expressing any residual air prior to closing.

Timely recognition of air entrapment is important to prevent early inappropriate shocks.[1,2] Device interrogation during pocket manipulation immediately after implantation can identify air entrapment by the presence of noise. In addition, a lateral chest radiograph is useful for timely recognition of air entrapment at the inferior and superior parasternal pockets (three-incisional technique) or at the inferior pocket (two-incisional technique). In case of air entrapment, temporary programming of a vector which avoids the affected electrode, or temporary inactivation of the S-ICD, may be considered. Subcutaneous air usually resorbs within a few days.

References

1. Yap SC, Bhagwandien RE, Szili-Torok T, Theuns DAMJ. Air entrapment causing early inappropriate shocks in a patient with a subcutaneous cardioverter-defibrillator. *Heart Rhythm Case Rep* 2015; 1: 157–8.
2. Zipes MM, Sauer WH, Varosy PD, Aleong RG, Nguyen DT. Inappropriate shocks due to subcutaneous air in a patient with a subcutaneous cardiac defibrillator. *Circ Arrhythm Electrophysiol* 2014; 7: 768–70.

Introduction to the case

A patient with idiopathic VF and resuscitated sudden death was referred after having been implanted with an S-ICD. At implantation, the S-ICD failed to defibrillate induced VF at 65 J and 80 J (Figure 50.1), which required external defibrillation. The chest X-ray directly after implantation is shown in Figure 50.2.

Figure 50.1 EGM of the S-ICD defibrillation test (the 65 J shock is shown on the bottom left-hand corner of the figure by ⚡, and the ineffective 80 J shock is not shown here)

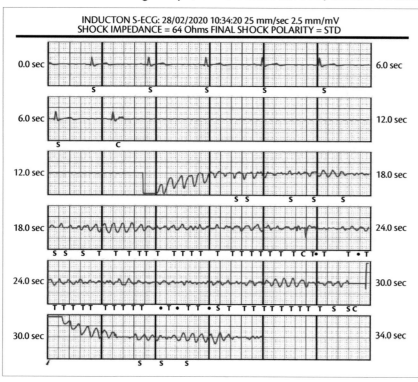

Question

Figure 50.2 Chest X-ray directly after S-ICD implantation

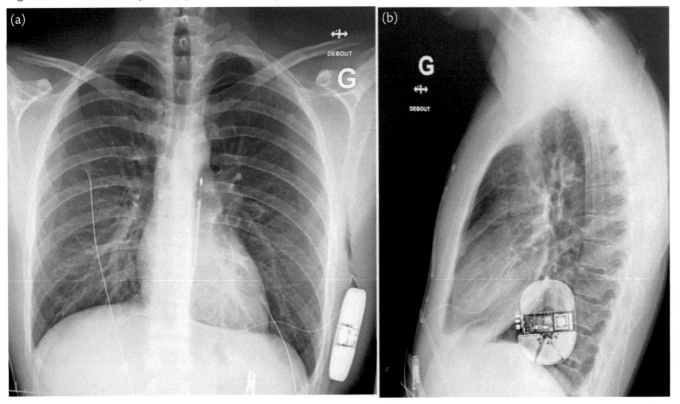

What is the most likely explanation for S-ICD shock failure?

A Air in the generator pocket

B Generator with suboptimal position

C Lead pin improperly inserted in the header

D Lead with suboptimal position

E Pneumothorax

Answer

D Lead with suboptimal position

Figure 50.3 Annotated tracing

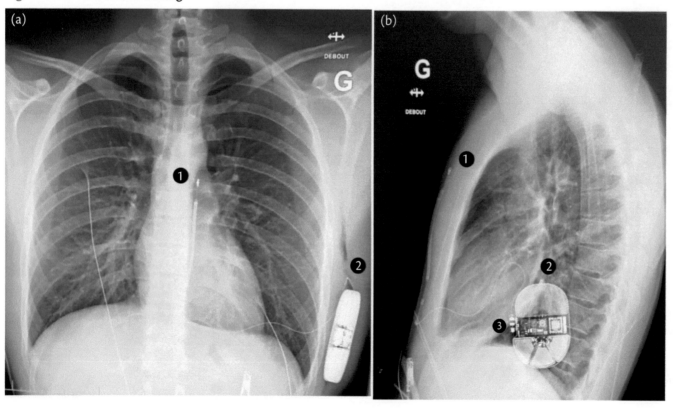

❶ In the posteroanterior X-ray (Figure 50.3a), the lead seems well positioned. However, the lateral chest X-ray (Figure 50.3b) shows the lead to be inadequately tunnelled, with a superficial course.

❷ The generator is well positioned adjacent to the cardiac apex in the posteroanterior chest X-ray (Figure 50.3a), and posterior to the midline in the lateral view (Figure 50.3b). There is some air in the pocket; however, the shock impedance was within normal limits and this factor is less likely than lead position to have affected the defibrillation threshold.

❸ The connector pin is well inserted in the header (the tip can be seen protruding), and the shock impedance was within normal limits, pointing against improper lead insertion in the generator.

Comments

Importance of subcutaneous implantable cardioverter defibrillator system position for treatment success

The lead was repositioned in a right parasternal position (to avoid merging of the new and initial tunnels) in a deeper plane with successful defibrillation at 65 J (15 J margin)—see Figure 50.4.

Figure 50.4 Repositioning of the S-ICD lead in a right parasternal position (a), with deeper tunnelling (b), and successful defibrillation at 65 J (c)

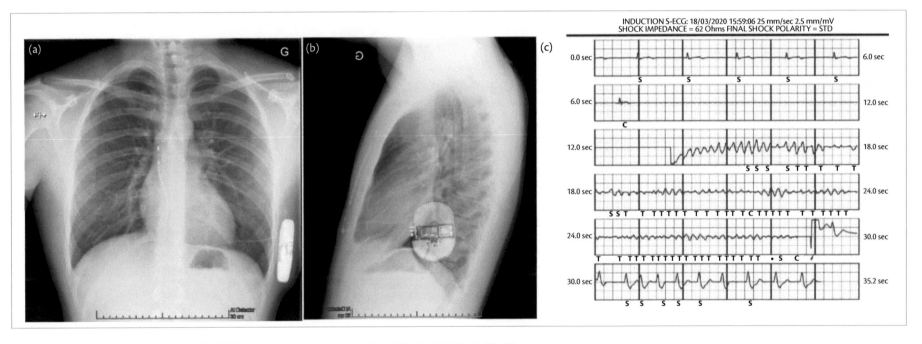

The PRAETORIAN study[1] identified different factors associated with high S-ICD defibrillation thresholds (Figure 50.5).

Figure 50.5 PRAETORIAN score for predicting defibrillation success with S-ICDs

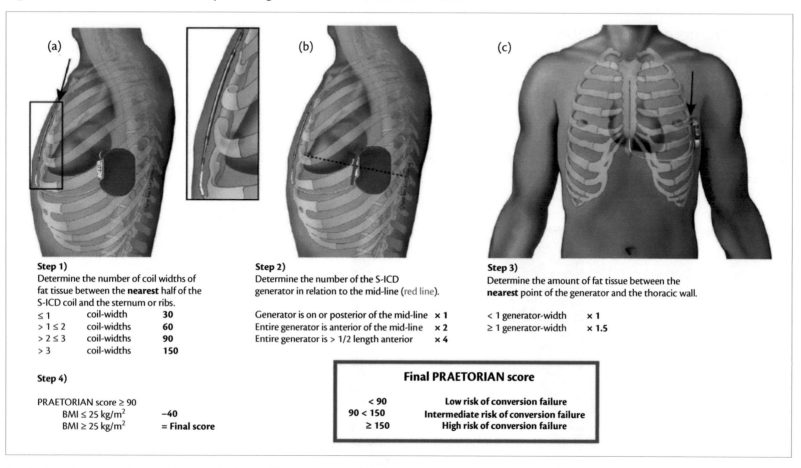

(a)   (b)   (c)

Step 1)
Determine the number of coil widths of
fat tissue between the **nearest** half of the
S-ICD coil and the sternum or ribs.

≤ 1	coil-width	30
> 1 ≤ 2	coil-widths	60
> 2 ≤ 3	coil-widths	90
> 3	coil-widths	150

Step 2)
Determine the number of the S-ICD
generator in relation to the mid-line (red line).

Generator is on or posterior of the mid-line	× 1
Entire generator is anterior of the mid-line	× 2
Entire generator is > 1/2 length anterior	× 4

Step 3)
Determine the amount of fat tissue between the
nearest point of the generator and the thoracic wall.

| < 1 generator-width | × 1 |
| ≥ 1 generator-width | × 1.5 |

Step 4)

PRAETORIAN score ≥ 90
BMI ≤ 25 kg/m^2 −40
BMI ≥ 25 kg/m^2 = Final score

Final PRAETORIAN score

< 90	Low risk of conversion failure
90 < 150	Intermediate risk of conversion failure
≥ 150	High risk of conversion failure

Reproduced from Quast ABE, Baalman SWE, Brouwer TF, Smeding L, Wilde AAM, Burke MC, Knops RE. A novel tool to evaluate the implant
position and predict defibrillation success of the subcutaneous implantable cardioverter-defibrillator: The PRAETORIAN score. *Heart Rhythm*. 2019
Mar;16(3):403–410. doi: 10.1016/j.hrthm.2018.09.029 with permission from Elsevier.

Reference

1. Quast ABE, Baalman SWE, Brouwer TF, et al. A novel tool to evaluate the implant position and predict defibrillation success
of the subcutaneous implantable cardioverter-defibrillator: the PRAETORIAN score. *Heart Rhythm* 2019; **16**: 403–10.

Section Three

CRT
Cases 51–70

Introduction to the case

A patient implanted with a CRT-D was managed by remote monitoring.

A transmission from the remote monitoring platform is shown in Figure 51.1.

Question

Figure 51.1 Report from the remote monitoring platform of the CRT-D patient

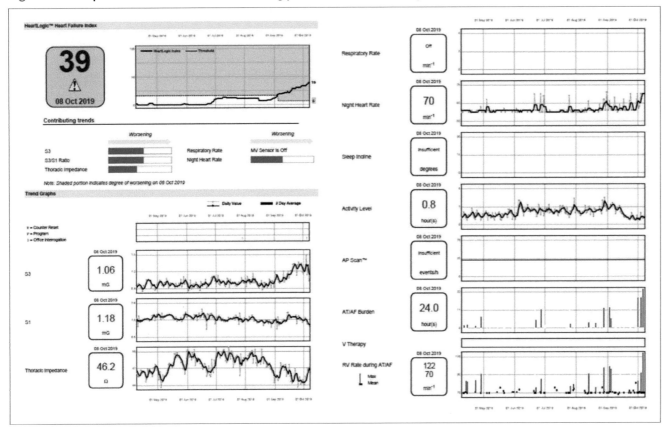

What would be the most appropriate next step?

A Admit the patient to the hospital

B Contact the patient to enquire about symptoms

C Inactivate remote monitoring

D Schedule a transmission in 2 weeks

E No action is necessary

Answer

B Contact the patient to enquire about symptoms

Figure 51.2 Annotated report

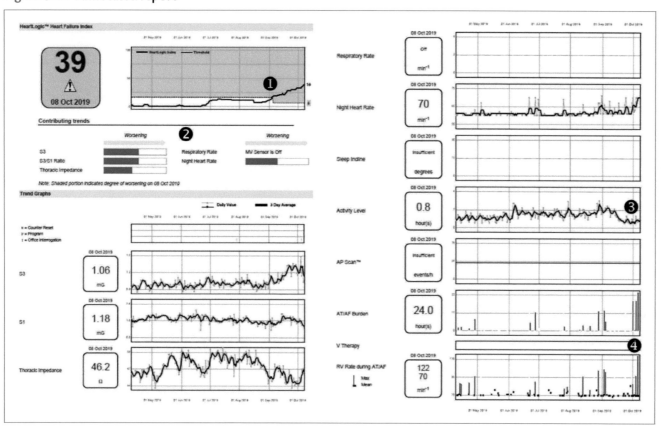

Figure 51.2 shows a report from the Boston Scientific HeartLogic diagnostic tool for monitoring heart failure.

❶ A crossing of the nominal HeartLogic composite index threshold of 16 (programmable 10–40) had triggered a yellow alert, with a continuing rise in the index. The threshold for recovery is automatically set to 6.

❷ The trends of the five contributing factors can be viewed here: S3 amplitude, S3/S1 amplitude, transthoracic impedance, respiratory rate and volume (inactivated), and nocturnal heart rate. Trends of these parameters, along with other diagnostic parameters, are also shown.

❸ Note the reduction in daily activity, which is synchronous with worsening of the contributing factors to the HeartLogic index.

❹ The patient has been experiencing an increase in AF burden (with an average ventricular rate of 70 bpm), which may be a consequence of worsening heart failure (note increase in S3, decrease in thoracic impedance, and reduction in daily activity which precede AF burden increase).

Overall, a worsening of the HeartLogic composite index is observed.

Comments

Utility of cardiac implantable electronic devices for monitoring heart failure

The patient was contacted and reported worsening heart failure symptoms with weight gain. He was referred to his cardiologist, who increased diuretic therapy, with clinical improvement.

In addition to monitoring heart rate and rhythm, cardiac implantable electronic devices are equipped with a number of sensors which can monitor daily activity (accelerometer), lung fluid (transthoracic impedance), respiratory rate and nocturnal apnoea (minute ventilation sensor), sleep incline, as well as S1 and S3 heart sounds (accelerometer). Algorithms integrate the different diagnostic parameters to yield indices which can be useful for managing patients remotely.

The Boston Scientific HeartLogic index with the nominal cut-off of 16 was evaluated in the Multisense study in CRT-D patients, and showed a 5.6% positive predictive value and >99% negative predictive value for heart failure admission or intravenous diuretic therapy over the following 45 days.[1]

The Medtronic TriageHF algorithm allows to risk stratify remote monitoring alerts to focus on the 10% of high-risk alerts (5.8% positive predictive value and 98% negative predictive value for cardiovascular hospitalizations over the following 30 days).[2]

Allied professionals are often first in line for managing remote monitoring alerts, and these algorithms can be useful in assisting them to risk stratify the alerts. However, it is as yet unknown whether these tools will reduce cardiovascular admissions by providing earlier detection of impending cardiac decompensation.

References

1. Boehmer JP, Hariharan R, Devecchi FG, et al. A multisensor algorithm predicts heart failure events in patients with implanted devices: results from the MultiSENSE Study. *JACC Heart Fail* 2017; **5**: 216–25.
2. Burri H, da Costa A, Quesada A, et al. Risk stratification of cardiovascular and heart failure hospitalizations using integrated device diagnostics in patients with a cardiac resynchronization therapy defibrillator. *Europace* 2018; **20**: e69–77.

Introduction to the case

A 50-year-old woman who had been implanted 5 years ago with a CRT-D, and had normalized her ejection fraction, presented at follow-up without any complaints. A tracing retrieved from the device memory is shown in Figure 52.1, which corresponded to when she was swimming.

Question

Figure 52.1 Event retrieved from the device memory

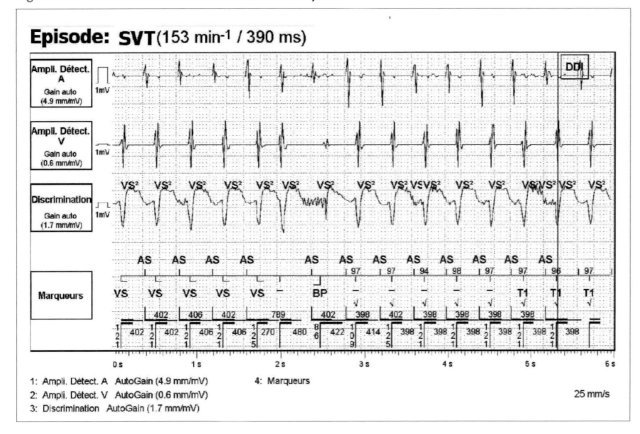

What action should be taken based upon this tracing?

A Check for fracture of the RV lead (RV coil)

B Decrease sensed AVI

C Decrease sensitivity of the discrimination channel

D Increase atrial sensitivity

E Increase MTR

Answer

E Increase MTR

Figure 52.2 Annotated tracing

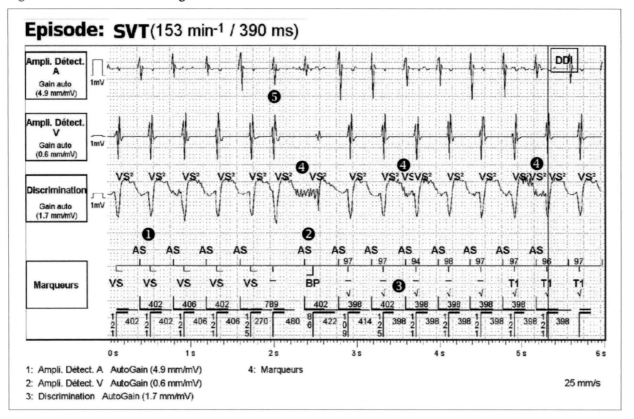

The patient lost biventricular pacing due to the sinus rate being faster than the MTR (Figure 52.2). Programmed parameters are not given in the question stem, but can be deduced from the tracing.

❶ Atrial events are not refractory but do not result in biventricular pacing due to intrinsic conduction occurring before pacing can be delivered (if there had been AVB, a pseudo-Wenckebach response would have been observed with ventricular pacing at the MTR).

❷ The programmed sensed AVI is 90 ms (86 ms is displayed due to measurement tolerance of the device processor, and can be considered as normal function). This is shorter than the intrinsic AVI of 121 ms, so shortening the sensed AVI would not solve the issue.

❸ Intervals which are <400 ms undergo the binning process, so the VT-1 zone is programmed at 150 bpm. In order to increase MTR to 150 bpm, the VT-1 limit needs to be increased to avoid interlock. Morphology discrimination is applied to all cycles during the event (with a '✓' indicating a match above the programmed threshold of 90%).

❹ Artefacts are observed on the discrimination channel and correspond to myopotentials (probably pectoral muscle contraction while swimming, due to the can being part of the sensing circuit). The artefacts are intermittently sensed by the channel (additional VS² markers) but do not incur a risk of inappropriate shock as they are not used for rate sensing (only the near-field events count). Sensitivity of the discrimination channel cannot be programmed.

❺ Ventricular premature beat with functional undersensing of the atrial signal due to blanking by the PVAB. Atrial sensitivity does not need to be increased.

Comments

Loss of cardiac resynchronization therapy delivery

Reduction in CRT delivery to <98%, <95%, and <90% is encountered in 40.7%, 22%, and 11.5% of patients respectively.[1] A number of causes for loss of CRT delivery are listed in Box 52.1, the most frequent one being atrial tachyarrhythmias.

Box 52.1 Causes for loss of CRT delivery

- Rapidly conducted AT/ atrial flutter/AF.

- Frequent ventricular premature beats.

- Idioventricular rhythm/junctional rhythm.

- Frequent conducted atrial premature beats.

- UTR programmed too low.

- AVI programmed too long.

- Increase in LV capture threshold (e.g. due to dislodgment or lead failure).

- Atrial undersensing.

- TWOS.

- Programming of a non-tracking mode—DDI(R) or VVI(R)—with sinus rhythm and AV conduction.

- Interlock with interventricular sensing (in devices with LV sensing).

- Automatic CRT optimization algorithms which require conducted beats (result in <2% of loss of CRT delivery).

Reference

1. Cheng A, Landman SR, Stadler RW. Reasons for loss of cardiac resynchronization therapy pacing: insights from 32 844 patients. *Circ Arrhythm Electrophysiol* 2012; 5: 884–8.

Introduction to the case

A patient with dilated cardiomyopathy, left ventricular ejection fraction (LVEF) of 25%, and NYHA class II heart failure under optimal medical therapy was implanted with a CRT-D. She presented with worsening dyspnoea 8 weeks after implantation. An ECG recorded during biventricular pacing and intrinsic rhythm is shown in Figure 53.1.

Question

Figure 53.1 ECG during biventricular pacing (a) and intrinsic rhythm (b)

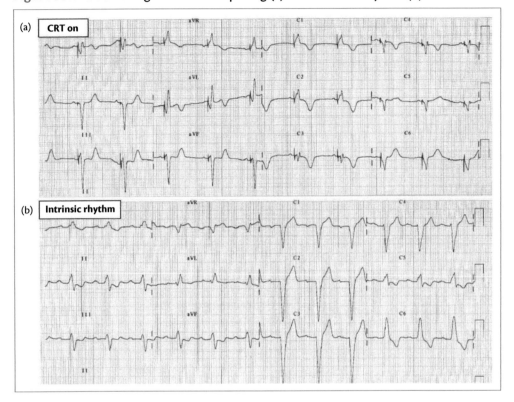

Which of the following reasons is the most likely for explaining non-response to CRT?

A Atrial undersensing

B AVI programmed too short

C Inappropriate patient selection

D Increase in LV capture threshold

E Increase in RV capture threshold

Answer

B AVI programmed too short

Figure 53.2 Annotated tracing

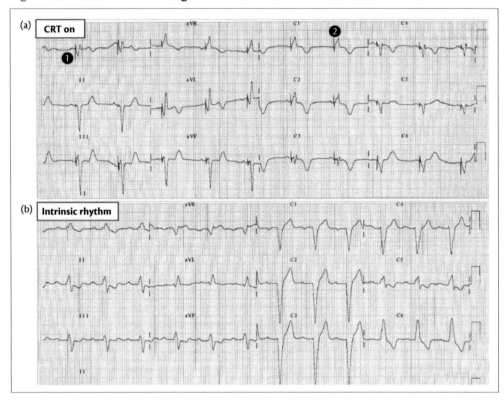

Although this patient has biventricular capture which may improve systolic function, the AVI is programmed too short, compromising diastolic function.

❶ The VP spike falls before the P-wave end (Figure 53.2), indicating that the AVI may be programmed too short.

❷ The R-wave in V1 and QR complex in lead I indicate effective LV capture. Loss of RV capture would have resulted in a wider QRS complex.

QRS morphology in intrinsic rhythm shows typical LBBB fulfilling the Strauss criteria (QRS duration >140 ms in men or 130 ms in women, QS or rS in leads V1 and V2, and mid-QRS notching or slurring in two or more consecutive leads V1, V2, V5, V6, I, and aVL[1]), which is predictive of response to CRT.[2] The clinical information given in the question stem also points towards appropriate patient selection.

Comments

Utility of the surface electrocardiogram for evaluating AV intervals for CRT

Although most patients may fare well with nominal CRT settings, a subset of patients benefit from optimization of AV and VV intervals. This is the case for patients with interatrial conduction delay, which is often induced by AP (Figure 53.3). Previous studies have shown that ventricular pacing should occur approximately 30–40 ms after the end of the P-wave.[3] An AVI which is programmed too short may truncate the mitral A-wave, resulting in suboptimal LV filling and increased left atrial pressure (see Volume 1, Case 60). The surface ECG can therefore provide useful clues for CRT optimization, not only in terms of QRS narrowing (which is associated with improved CRT response[4,5]) and optimizing VV intervals due to LV latency (see Volume 1, Case 62), but also in terms of AV timing. This premise forms the basis AV optimization algorithms which measure P-wave duration on unipolar signals of the atrial lead in some CRT devices (Medtronic).

References

1. Strauss DG, Selvester RH, Wagner GS. Defining left bundle branch block in the era of cardiac resynchronization therapy. *Am J Cardiol* 2011; **107**: 927–34.
2. van Stipdonk AMW, Hoogland R, Ter Horst I, et al. Evaluating electrocardiography-based identification of cardiac resynchronization therapy responders beyond current left bundle branch block definitions. *JACC Clin Electrophysiol* 2020; **6**: 193–203.
3. Jones RC, Svinarich T, Rubin A, et al. Optimal atrioventricular delay in CRT patients can be approximated using surface electrocardiography and device electrograms. *J Cardiovasc Electrophysiol* 2010; **21**: 1226–32.
4. Trucco E, Tolosana JM, Arbelo E, et al. Improvement of reverse remodeling using electrocardiogram fusion-optimized intervals in cardiac resynchronization therapy: a randomized study. *JACC Clin Electrophysiol* 2018; **4**: 181–9.
5. Jastrzębski M, Baranchuk A, Fijorek K, et al. Cardiac resynchronization therapy-induced acute shortening of QRS duration predicts long-term mortality only in patients with left bundle branch block. *Europace* 2019; **21**: 281–9.

Figure 53.3 Marked interatrial conduction delay in a patient requiring atrial pacing, with a P-wave duration of 280 ms (normal <120 ms), best seen in lead II

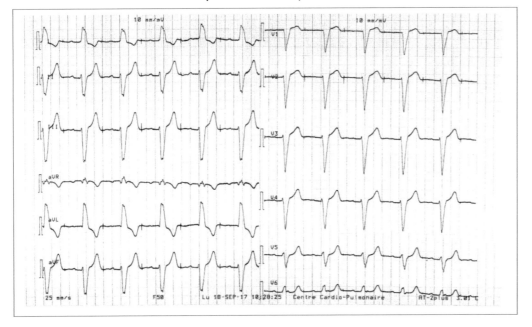

Introduction to the case

A patient with dilated cardiomyopathy and LBBB implanted with a CRT-D was seen at follow-up. The patient had no complaints. Percentage of ventricular pacing was 98% (with LV pacing only). During in-office follow-up, the ECG shown in Figure 54.1 was observed.

Question

Figure 54.1 ECGs recorded during in-office follow-up

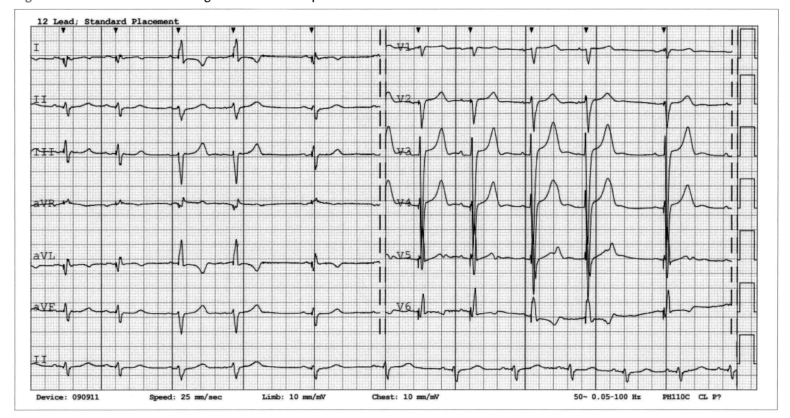

What is the reason for the transient change in QRS morphology?

A Atrial ectopic beats

B Atrial undersensing

C AV hysteresis

D CRT optimization algorithm

E Elevation in LV capture threshold

Answer

A Atrial ectopic beats

Figure 54.2 Annotated tracing

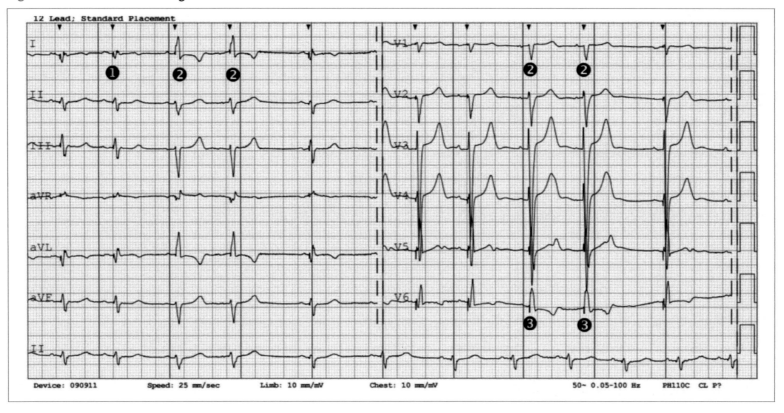

❶ Sinus rhythm with LV fusion pacing is visible (Figure 54.2), with a relatively narrow QRS complex (note the Q-waves in lead I suggestive of LV capture)

❷ These two cycles show atrial ectopic beats from two different foci (note the difference in P-wave morphology, visible in lead I). The QRS morphology is slightly wider, resembling more a LBB pattern due to less contribution of LV capture. Some degree of capture is present as the QRS is still relatively narrow (approximately 120 ms).

❸ A ventricular pacing spike is visible, indicating that the atrial beats had been sensed and tracked.

Comments

Effect of atrial ectopic beats on cardiac resynchronization therapy delivery

Conducted atrial premature beats may result in loss of CRT if they fall in the PVARP (and are thereby not tracked) or due to limitation of the UTR.

Ectopic beats may also result in loss of ventricular pacing if the intrinsic PR interval is shortened due to the ectopy originating close to the AVN (as with the first atrial premature beat in this case example). Alternatively, if sensing occurs late in the right atrial lead (e.g. due to a left atrial ectopic beat), the programmed sensed AV delay may be too long (Figure 54.3).

Figure 54.3 Intrinsic sensed AVIs (yellow arrows) resulting from sinus rhythm (green), atrial ectopy close to the AVN (blue) with a short PR interval, and atrial ectopy originating far from the right atrial lead (red) with delayed sensing by the device. The programmed AV delays are depicted in orange. In sinus rhythm, biventricular pacing will result from the programmed AV delay being shorter than the sensed intrinsic AV delay, whereas with ectopic rhythm, intrinsic conduction will result

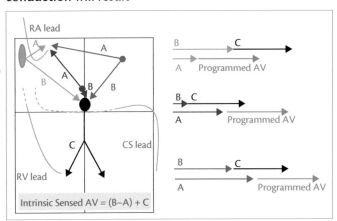

Introduction to the case

A patient with a CRT-D was seen at follow-up. The patient did not have any complaints. Biventricular pacing was delivered in 97% of the time, with 3% VS events. There were no VT/VF episodes (VT monitor zone 150–188 bpm, fast VT zone 188–240 bpm, VF zone >240 bpm). The tracing shown in Figure 55.1 was retrieved from the device memory as a 'ventricular sensing episode' which had lasted for 3 minutes.

Question

Figure 55.1 Event retrieved from the device memory (only marker intervals are available)

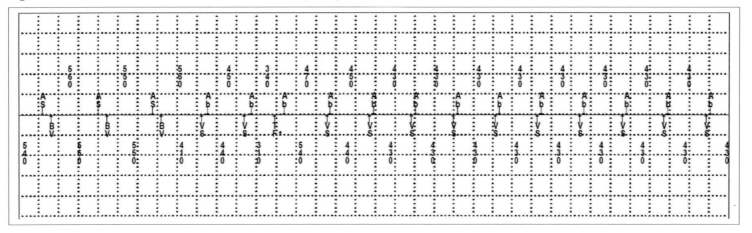

What do you observe?

A AT

B AVNRT

C AVRT

D VT

E None of the above

Answer

D VT

Figure 55.2 Annotated tracing

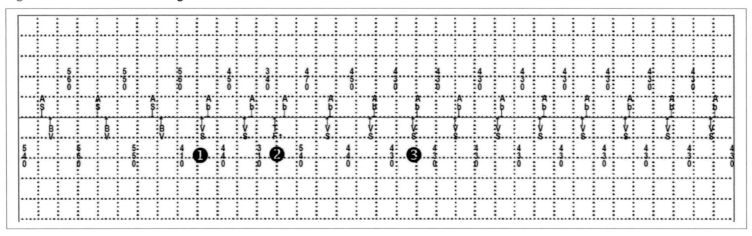

❶ The arrhythmia is initiated by a ventricular event (Figure 55.2). This pleads against AT or typical AVNRT.

❷ The short–long VV sequence (310–540 ms) precedes the short–long AA sequence (340–470 ms). This also points against AT. With the short VV sequence (310 ms), note the slight prolongation of the VA interval due to decremental conduction (which points against retrograde conduction via an accessory pathway and AVRT).

❸ The VT stabilizes at a cycle length of 430 ms. This is slower than the VT detection zone and is therefore not classified as such.

Comments

Ventricular sensed events in biventricular devices

Sustained VS events are recorded in some biventricular devices and can result from a variety of causes listed in Box 55.1.

Box 55.1 Causes of sustained VS events in biventricular devices

- Atrial undersensing.

- Sinus tachycardia above the UTR.

- Conducted atrial arrhythmias (falling below the mode switch rate).

- AVNRT.

- Unduly long programmed AVI.

- Atrial ectopic rhythm (e.g. near coronary sinus ostium) with short PR interval.

- Accelerated ventricular rhythm/slow ventricular tachycardia.

In this example, the short (50 ms) VA interval probably resulted from a left-sided VT, with delayed detection in the RV. This can masquerade as typical AVNRT. Far-field (e.g. can to coil) EGMs are useful if available, as the VA interval should be measured from QRS onset.

The question arises regarding management of slow VTs discovered fortuitously or detected in monitoring zones. Decisions must be made on a case-by-case basis and should take into account factors such as related symptoms, ventricular function, duration of the arrhythmia, and arrhythmic substrate. Antiarrhythmic medication, ablation, or programming of ICD therapy (including ATP only in some instances) are options.

Introduction to the case

A 67-year-old patient with a CRT-D was seen at follow-up. The patient complained of breathlessness upon exertion. Lead testing was normal. The patient underwent a treadmill test. A real-time EGM taken during the test is shown in Figure 56.1.

Question

Figure 56.1 Device EGM

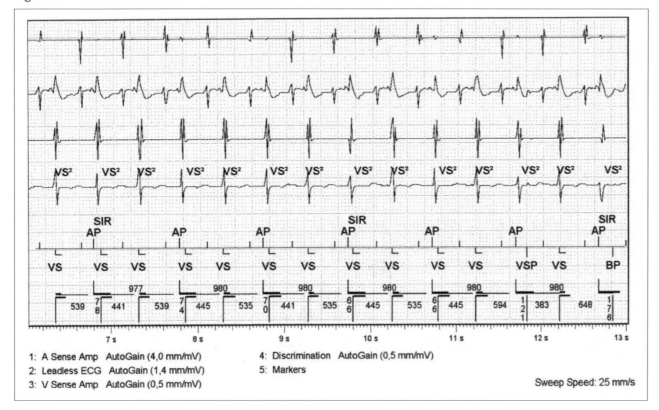

What programming change should be made?

A Decrease AV delay

B Decrease PVARP

C Increase atrial sensitivity

D Increase PVAB

E Increase slope of rate response

Answer

B Decrease PVARP

Figure 56.2 Annotated EGM

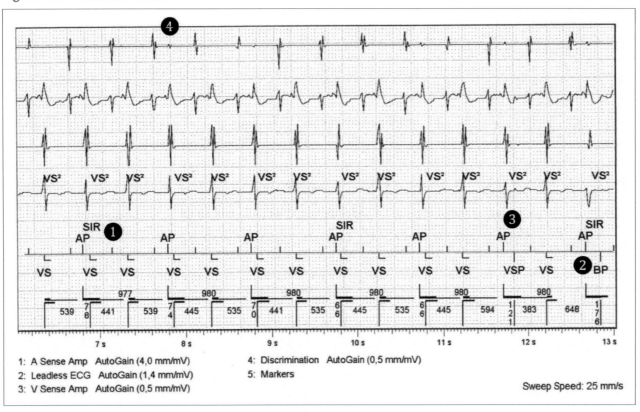

The EGM in Figure 56.2 shows sinus tachycardia at 130 bpm with intrinsic AV conduction and non-delivery of biventricular pacing. This is due to all AS events falling in the long programmed PVARP (set to 400 ms according to the markers) and also heart rate being above the UTR (see below). Although device settings are not disclosed in this case, several parameters can be deduced from the information given in the tracing.

❶ All intrinsic atrial cycles are sensed as AR events (as shown by the markers) as they fall in the PVARP. Increasing atrial sensitivity will not solve this issue.

❷ The paced AV delay is set to 180 ms (the 176 ms marker is due to tolerance of the device clock). The MTR is therefore limited to 103 (60,000/580) bpm due to limitation of the total AR period = AVI + PVARP = 180 + 400 = 580 ms. The sinus rate is therefore faster than the MTR. The device is pacing at the sensor indicated rate (SIR) of 61 bpm (AP–AP intervals of 980 ms). There does not appear to be a need for DDDR pacing as the patient does not seem to have chronotropic insufficiency.

❸ Ventricular safety pacing occurs 120 ms after AP due to VS in the ventricular safety pacing window (of 64 ms in this device). All other VS events following AP cycles fall out of the ventricular safety pacing window.

❹ AP artefacts on the atrial channel, which are not to be confounded with FFRWs, as they are only visible after AP cycles.

Comments

Non-delivery of cardiac resynchronization therapy due to long post-ventricular atrial refractory period and limited upper tracking rate

A long PVARP may be intentionally programmed or result from automatic post-PVC PVARP extension by the device, in order to avoid endless loop tachycardia. This can, however, result in non-tracking of sinus tachycardia, as in this case. As with a long AVI, a long PVARP also limits the UTR. Automatic PVARP and AVIs (which shorten with increasing rates) are usually programmed to be able to increase the UTR and maintain biventricular pacing at exercise. A common mistake is to leave the UTR at default settings, and not adapt this parameter to the patient's requirements (which should take into account the patient's age and physical activity).

Post-PVC PVARP extension will depend on the definition of a PVC by the device, which differs between manufacturers. With Abbott, a PVC is defined as a VS event which is not preceded by an AP or AS event, including refractory sense if the AR–VS interval is >280 ms (>350 ms for Biotronik). In the present case, AR–VS intervals were about 180 ms, and post-PVC PVARP extension does not explain the long PVARP. With Medtronic, post-PVC PVARP extension is only triggered for a VS event (refractory or non-refractory) without an intervening atrial event (pace, sense, or refractory sense).

Introduction to the case

A patient complained of persistent heart failure symptoms 6 months after CRT implantation. Device follow-up showed excellent capture thresholds with 99% VP and no sustained arrhythmias. The paced AVI had been programmed at the default value of 130 ms. An echocardiogram was performed, and the transmitral pulsed-wave Doppler flow is shown in Figure 57.1.

Question

Figure 57.1 Transmitral pulsed-wave Doppler with different programmed AVIs

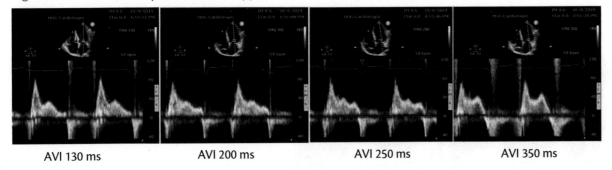

| AVI 130 ms | AVI 200 ms | AVI 250 ms | AVI 350 ms |

How should the AVI be programmed?

A 130 ms

B 200 ms

C 250 ms

D 350 ms

E AVI programming will not affect response in this case

Answer

C 250 ms

Figure 57.2 Annotated figure

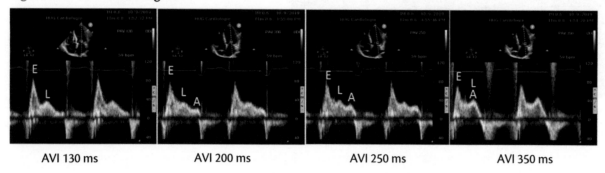

AVI 130 ms   AVI 200 ms   AVI 250 ms   AVI 350 ms

At the programmed AVI of 130 ms, the E-wave is easily recognizable (Figure 57.2), followed by a lower-velocity broad waveform which may be mistaken as being the A-wave but is in fact the late ('L') wave. At 250 ms, the A-wave is visible, and contributes to LV filling. This A-wave is slightly truncated at 200 ms, which is suboptimal. It is fused with the A-wave at 350 ms. Such a long AVI will limit the UTR and may also result in pseudo-fusion (although the paced QRS complex looks similar with all these settings in the single displayed lead and should be confirmed with a 12-lead ECG).

Comments

Transmitral flow patterns with varying programmed atrioventricular delays

Although there is no evidence that routine echographic optimization of AV delays improves clinical outcome, it may be useful in a subset of patients where default or automatic settings may be suboptimal. The most salient feature of a suboptimal AV interval is truncation of the A-wave, which compromises LV filling (see Volume 1, Case 60). The AV delay may be optimized by the iterative method, whereby a value about 40 ms shorter than the AS/AP–VS interval is initially programmed and the transmitral flow pattern is evaluated with decrementing values (10–20 ms) of the programmed AV delay, until A-wave truncation is observed.

In this example, an L-wave is observed, which may be mistaken for the A-wave. L-waves are seen in diastolic dysfunction and are independent of atrial contraction (i.e. they may also be observed in patients in AF).[1,2] The transmitral flow in intrinsic rhythm is shown in Figure 57.3 (note that the QRS complex is different compared to paced rhythm in Figure 57.2, even at a programmed delay of 350 ms).

Figure 57.3 Transmitral flow pattern in intrinsic rhythm showing E-, L-, and A-waves

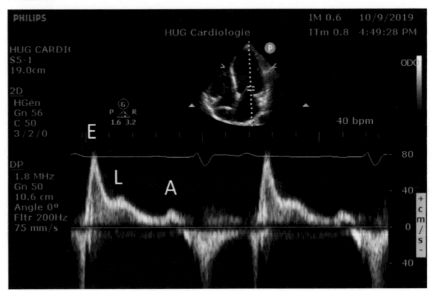

References

1. Morisawa D, Ohno Y, Ohta Y, et al. Serial changes of L wave according to heart rates in a heart failure patient with persistent atrial fibrillation. *J Cardiol Cases* 2019; **20**: 213–17.
2. Kim SA, Son J, Shim CY, Choi EY, Ha JW. Long-term outcome of patients with triphasic mitral flow with a mid-diastolic L wave: prognostic role of left atrial volume and N-terminal pro-brain natriuretic peptide. *Int J Cardiovasc Imaging* 2017; **33**: 1377–84.

Introduction to the case

A patient with a cardiac resynchronization therapy pacemaker (CRT-P) presented to the out-patient clinic for routine device follow-up. The patient's ECG is shown in Figure 58.1.

Question

Figure 58.1 ECG (precordial leads) during in-office CRT-P follow-up

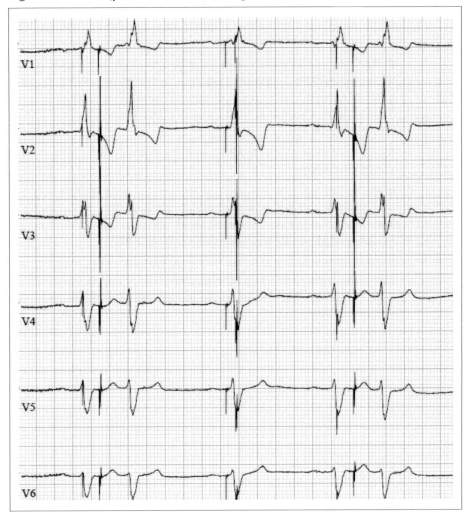

What is the most appropriate first management step?

A Increase atrial sensitivity

B Increase output of the LV lead

C Increase output of the RV lead

D Increase PVAB

E Increase ventricular sensitivity

Answer

A Increase atrial sensitivity

Figure 58.2 Annotated ECG

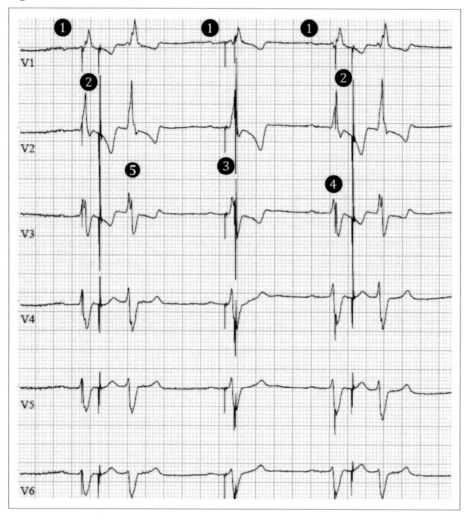

The ECG in Figure 58.2 displays atrial undersensing with non-delivery of CRT.

❶ The sinus P-waves are not sensed. These P-waves are conducted with a prolonged PR interval of approximately 240 ms.

❷ AP on the conducted QRS complex, with 'pseudo-pseudo-fusion' and a paced AVI of 180 ms. Intrinsic QRS complexes are not sensed as they fall in the PAVB. The ventricular spike falls during the T-wave and is not captured due to the myocardium being refractory. Note that the ventricular spike has two discrete components, due to a very short interventricular delay.

❸ Shortened paced AVI due to AP followed by ventricular sensing in the ventricular safety pacing window.

❹ The VA interval can be measured from this AP spike to the preceding ventricular spike. Note that AP falls considerably late after QRS onset (about 80 ms), implying that this ventricular event was not yet sensed on the ventricular channel. This is explained by delayed sensing by the RV lead due to the underlying RBBB.

❺ Intrinsic QRS complex, due either to a conducted atrial premature beat (hidden in the T-wave) or junctional ectopy. This ventricular event is properly sensed, as it resets the VA interval (with pacing at 50 bpm) Note the slight change in QRS morphology due to aberrant conduction.

Comments

Atrial undersensing as a cause for non-delivery of biventricular pacing

Proper atrial sensing is essential for tracking of sinus rhythm and delivery of biventricular pacing. It is also important for detection of supraventricular arrhythmias (which are prevalent in this patient population) and proper rhythm discrimination of ICDs.

This case also illustrates the potential danger of programming long paced AVIs. In the event of atrial pacing which is simultaneous to an intrinsic QRS complex (either due to a ventricular premature beat or a conducted beat after atrial undersensing, as in this case), functional ventricular undersensing will occur due to the PAVB. Ventricular pacing may then be delivered in the vulnerable part of the T-wave, which may be proarrhythmic (see Volume 1, Cases 11 and 30).

Introduction to the case

A patient with a CRT-P device was seen at device follow-up. He did not have any complaints. An EGM retrieved from the device memory is shown in Figure 59.1.

Question

Figure 59.1 Retrieved EGM of AMS episode

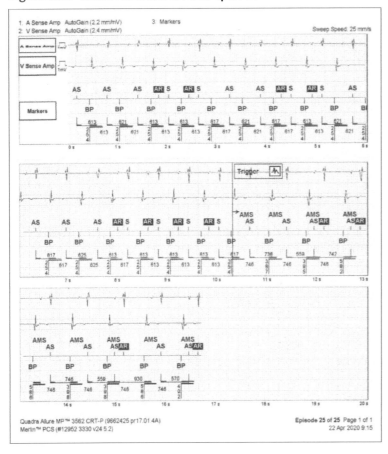

What is the most appropriate action?

A Decrease atrial sensitivity

B Decrease AMS rate

C Increase PVAB

D Increase PVARP

E No action is needed

Answer

C Increase PVAB

Figure 59.2 Annotated tracing

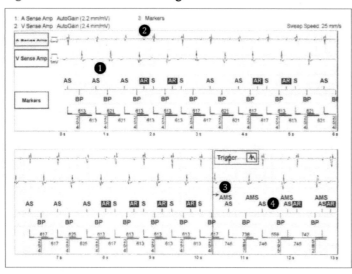

FFRW oversensing by the atrial channel led to inappropriate mode switch (Figure 59.2).

❶ DDD pacing with a long programmed sensed AVI of 250 ms (the displayed interval of 254 ms is due to the device clock), which had been optimized under echocardiography to avoid truncating the mitral A-wave.

❷ A small FFRW is observed on the atrial channel and is sensed in the PVARP (as indicated by the corresponding AR marker). FFRW oversensing is intermittent thereafter.

❸ Sufficient AR events have occurred for the AMS criteria to have been fulfilled and the device switches from DDD to a DDIR pacing mode with a lower rate of 80 bpm (or 750 ms pacing interval, with the displayed biventricular paced (BP)–BP interval of 746 ms being due to allowance of the device clock). This is not the sensor-driven rate, otherwise an 'SIR' ('sensor-indicated rate') marker would have been displayed.

❹ The patient has AVB. Abbott devices do not have a PVARP during mode switching, explaining why the FFRWs are now labelled 'AS' and not 'AR'.

Comments

Importance of far-field R-wave oversensing in cardiac resynchronization therapy

FFRW oversensing is favoured if the signal is of high amplitude (e.g. due to the atrial lead being implanted at the tip of the RA appendage, which overlies the RV outflow tract) and/or if the signal occurs late (after the PVAB), that is, in case the intrinsic or paced QRS is wide. It may also occur in the setting of RBBB, as the FFRW may be sensed in the atrial channel *before* delayed near-field sensing by the RV lead (in this instance, the PVAB is ineffective, and only a reduction in atrial sensitivity will solve the issue —see Volume 1, Case 10).

The issue is usually easily solved by prolonging the PVAB. An alternative is to decrease atrial sensitivity, but this may result in atrial undersensing. It is important to observe the atrial signal at implantation and to reposition the lead in a more anterior position if a large FFRW is seen. Some atrial leads have short electrode spacing, which reduces far-field ventricular signals.

Inappropriate mode switch resulting from FFRWs will lead to non-tracking of sinus rhythm and loss of biventricular pacing. This was not an issue in the current case due to AVB, but nevertheless resulted in AV dyssynchrony with a 'P on T' phenomenon, which may have compromised pump function (see Volume 1, Case 14).

Introduction to the case

A 59-year-old man with non-compaction cardiomyopathy and symptomatic heart failure had been implanted with a CRT-D. He presented for regular follow-up and did not report any complaints. An event classified as AMS was retrieved from the device memory and is shown in Figure 60.1. The device settings are shown in Table 60.1.

Table 60.1 Device settings

Tachycardia		
Zone	VT-1	VF
Rate (bpm/ms)	181/330	230/260
Detection	100	40
Discrimination	On	
Therapy	ATP + shocks	Shocks
Bradycardia		
Mode	DDDR	
Base rate	60 bpm	
MTR	150 bpm	
Maximum sensor rate	140 bpm	
Paced AV delay	150 ms	
Sensed AV delay	120 ms	
VP	Simultaneous	
PVARP	275 ms	
AT/AF detection rate	180 bpm	

Question

Figure 60.1 EGM of the AMS episode

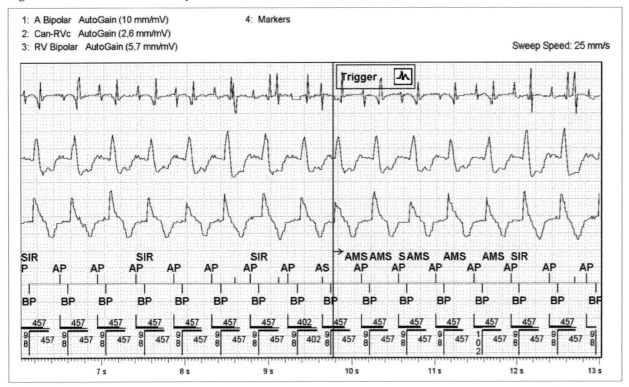

What is the cause of the atrial high-rate episode?

A Atrial bigeminy

B Atrial flutter

C Atrial non-capture

D FFRW oversensing

E Retrograde conducted atrial activity

Answer

C Atrial non-capture

Figure 60.2 Annotated EGM

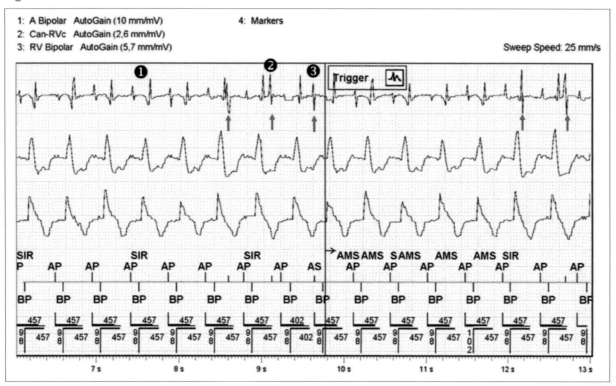

❶ The small signals are the AP artefacts (Figure 60.2). The rhythm is sensor driven (SIR) at about 130 bpm. The larger signals are caused by FFRWs which fall in the PVAB (no annotation on the marker channel). There is therefore no FFRW oversensing. Note the stable interval between biventricular paced ('BP') and FFRW on the atrial EGM which is about 130 ms.

❷ Intrinsic atrial activity (sinus tachycardia at about 110 bpm) is intermittently visible, caused by atrial non-capture, and is indicated by the red arrows. The first two and last events fall in the PVARP (note the vertical short upward lines in the marker channel). The

third event falls outside the PVARP and is denoted by AS and triggers an AVI. The fourth event falls in the PVAB and is synchronous with the FFRW. Note that these events are asynchronous with the paced rhythm and are therefore not due to retrograde conduction.

❸ Following the AS events occurring in addition to AP, the atrial mode switch rate of 180 bpm is exceeded and mode switch is triggered, with pacing in the DDIR mode. In this older device, AP–AR intervals are counted towards the filtered atrial rate interval (FARI)—see Case 8 for mode switch criteria.

Comments

Inappropriate mode switch

By far the most common reason for inappropriate mode switch is FFRW oversensing. The problem can usually be solved by increasing the PVAB, as in Case 59. An issue, however, is patients with RBBB, in whom FFRW may occur *before* RV sensing (the PVAB in this instance is ineffective—see Volume 1, Case 10).

Other causes of inappropriate mode switch are atrial non-capture (as in the present example), RNRVAS, noise (due to EMI or lead fracture), and P-wave double counting in case of fragmented atrial potentials.[1]

Reference

1. Ganiere V, Cassagneau R, Burri H, Defaye P. Inappropriate mode switch consecutive to P-wave double counting. *Europace* 2011; **13**: 1795–6.

Introduction to the case

A 66-year-old man with a CRT-D for secondary prevention of sudden cardiac death presented for routine follow-up. He had no complaints. An event classified as AF was retrieved from the device memory and is shown in Figure 61.1. The device settings are shown in Table 61.1.

Table 61.1 Device settings

Tachycardia			
Zone	**VT-1**	**VT-2**	**VF**
Rate (bpm/ms)	136/440	169/355	230/260
Detection	24	20	18
Discrimination	On	On	
Therapy	ATP	ATP + shocks	shocks
Bradycardia			
Mode	DDDR		
Base rate	70 bpm		
MTR	110 bpm		
Maximum sensor rate	125 bpm		
Paced AV delay	130 ms		
Sensed AV delay	100 ms		
VP	LV – 20 ms		
PVARP	275 ms		
Shortest PVARP	225 ms		
AT/AF detection rate	180 bpm		

Question

Figure 61.1 EGM of the retrieved episode

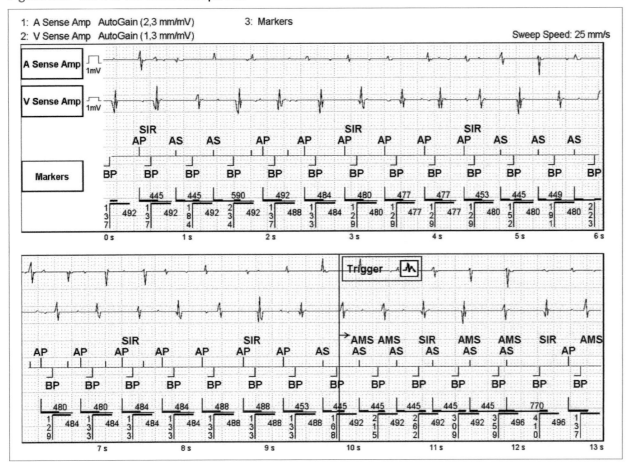

What triggers the AMS?

A AF

B Competition between sinus tachycardia and sensor-driven rate

C FFRW oversensing

D Endless loop tachycardia

E RNRVAS

Answer

B Competition between sinus tachycardia and sensor-driven rate

Figure 61.2 Annotated EGM of the retrieved episode

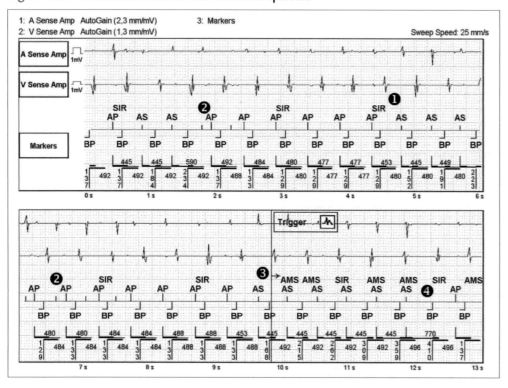

❶ The sinus rate is approximately 135 bpm (Figure 61.2), which is faster than the MTR or 110 bpm. This results in a progressive prolongation of sensed AV delay due to upper rate behaviour (pseudo-Wenckebach response).

❷ Sinus beats are detected in the PVARP (| markers) which is initiated by a prolonged AVI (last cycle of the top strip), without triggering of an AVI. Atrial pacing occurs at the SIR. Repetition of ARS and AP sequences may at first sight resemble RNRVAS. However, with RNRVAS, the VP–ARS intervals are relatively constant due to retrograde conduction (whereas here they shorten). The AR events are due to sinus tachycardia, and not due to FFRW oversensing.

❸ AMS is triggered which is above the programmed AT detection rate of 180 bpm. The filtered atrial rate interval had already fallen below the ATDI beforehand, due to the short AR–AP intervals (which are taken into account in this older device), but AMS is only triggered once an AS event is detected.

❹ The brady mode during AMS is DDIR which is a non-tracking mode. In Abbott devices, there is no PVARP during AMS (only PVAB), which explains why the atrial events are labelled as AS and not AR events.

Comments

Upper tracking rate, sensor rate, and mode switch

The sensor rate should be programmed equal or slightly below (e.g. −10 bpm) to the UTR, otherwise asynchronous VP may result. This may have adverse haemodynamic consequences. Another issue is inappropriate mode switch, as in the present case.

Rate response should only be programmed in case of chronotropic insufficiency, especially in CRT patients in whom AS is preferable to pacing due to avoidance of interatrial conduction delay and left AV dyssynchrony.[1]

Reference

1. Mullens W, Auricchio A, Martens P, et al. Optimized implementation of cardiac resynchronization therapy—a call for action for referral and optimization of care. *Eur J Heart Fail* 2020; **22**: 2349–69.

Introduction to the case

A 67-year-old man with ischaemic cardiopathy, NYHA class II
heart failure, and a wide QRS complex received a CRT-D
for primary prevention of sudden cardiac death. An event
classified as non-sustained RV oversensing was transmitted
by remote monitoring and is shown in Figure 62.1. Device
settings are shown in Table 62.1.

Table 62.1 Device settings

Tachycardia			
Zone	VT-1	VT-2	VF
Rate (bpm/ms)	166/360	187/320	230/260
Detection	30	30	20
Discrimination	On	On	
Therapy	Monitor	ATP + shocks	Shocks
Bradycardia			
Mode	DDD		
Base rate	60 bpm		
MTR	130 bpm		
Paced AV delay	225 ms		
Shortest AV delay	180 ms		
VP	LV – 60 ms		
PVARP	275 ms		

Question

Figure 62.1 EGM of the transmitted episode of non-sustained RV oversensing

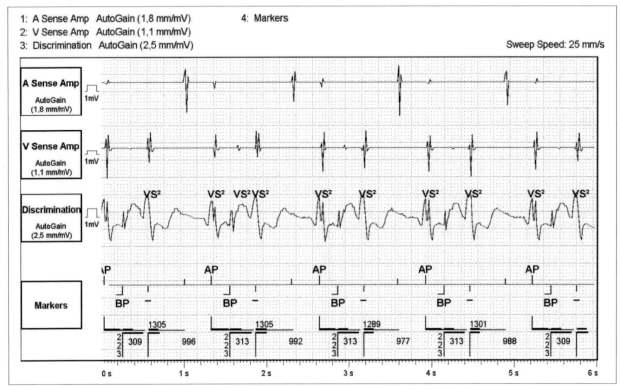

What is your diagnosis?

A Atrial bigeminy

B Loss of RV capture with LV-only capture

C FFRW oversensing

D TWOS

E Ventricular bigeminy

Answer

E Ventricular bigeminy

Figure 62.2 Annotated EGM of the transmitted episode

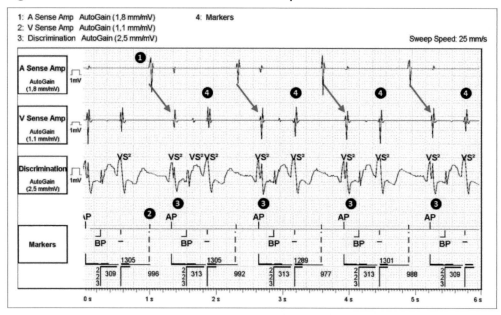

The EGM in Figure 62.2 shows normal device behaviour during ventricular bigeminy.

❶ High- and low-amplitude signals are visible on the atrial EGM. The high-amplitude signals are intrinsic atrial events (sinus rhythm) and the low-amplitude signals correspond to AP events. Sinus rhythm is conducted to the ventricle (red arrows), but the R-wave is not sensed due to simultaneous AP (functional undersensing due to cross-chamber blanking in the PAVB). It is, however, detected in the discrimination channel (VS² marker).

❷ The preceding VS event is detected as a PVC, which results in an extended PVARP of 475 ms (in order to avoid endless loop tachycardia). The intrinsic atrial event is detected in the prolonged PVARP (red dashed line) and therefore does not trigger an AVI.

❸ The PVC response algorithm of Abbott devices not only prolongs the PVARP, but also triggers AP at 330 ms after the refractory sensed atrial event. The AP event starts an AV timer and biventricular pacing is delivered after 223 ms.

❹ The ventricular EGM shows a repetitive group of three amplitude signals. The first high-amplitude signal corresponds to the intrinsic conducted ventricular event (which is not sensed). The second signal, of low amplitude, corresponds to the sequential biventricular pacing artefact, without evidence of capture on the far-field discrimination channel (due to the ventricular myocardial being refractory). The third signal, of high amplitude, corresponds to a PVC (note the different QRS morphology compared to the conducted beat).

Comments

Utility of far-field electrogram recordings

This case illustrates the importance of carefully analysing all available device channels to elucidate puzzling tracings. When available, far-field channels (such as the discrimination channel in this example, intended for detecting RV oversensing due to lead fracture), are very useful to use as surrogates of ECGs. They allow easier evaluation of QRS morphology than the bipolar signal recorded by the ventricular lead. They also allow QRS onset to be more readily appreciated, which can be useful for evaluating delay from VP, as well as VA intervals in case of 1:1 tachycardias (e.g. in case AVNRT is suspected).

Introduction to the case

A patient with dilated cardiomyopathy was implanted with a CRT-D. He presented with dyspnoea. The device memory indicated 88% biventricular pacing. Device programming is shown in Table 63.1. Capture thresholds were within usual limits. An ECG was recording during follow-up and is displayed in Figure 63.1. A real-time EGM is shown in Figure 63.2.

Table 63.1 Device programming

Bradycardia parameters	
Mode	DDD
Lower/upper rate	50/130
AV delay sensed/paced	100/130
Biventricular pacing	AdaptivCRT Bi-V and LV
Atrial lead	
Programmed output	2 V @ 0.4 ms
Pace polarity	Bipolar
Programmed sensitivity	0.45 mV
Sense polarity	Bipolar
PVARP	Auto (minimum 250 ms)
Right ventricular lead	
Programmed output	2 V @ 0.4 ms
Pace polarity	Bipolar
Programmed sensitivity	0.45 mV
Sense polarity	True bipolar (RV tip to RV ring)
Ventricular blanking post VP	230 ms
Ventricular blanking post VS	120 ms

Left ventricular lead	
Programmed output	3 V @ 1 ms
Pace polarity	Extended bipolar (LV2 to RV coil)
Tachycardia parameters	
Slow VT zone (monitor only)	140–194 bpm (NID 40 intervals)
Fast VT zone via VF (ATP + shocks)	194–240 bpm (30/40 intervals)
VF zone (ATP during charge, 6× shocks)	>240 bpm (30/40 intervals)

Bi-V, biventricular.

Figure 63.1 ECG recorded during follow-up

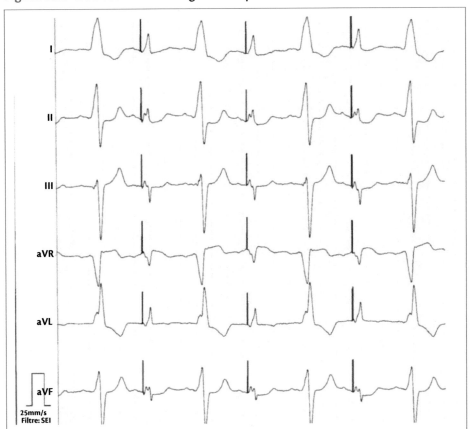

25mm/s
Filtre: SEI

Question

Figure 63.2 Real-time EGM during device follow-up

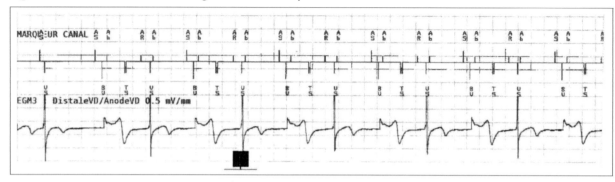

How can the issue be best solved?

A   Activate TWOS algorithm

B   Inactivate post-PVC PVARP extension

C   Increase atrial sensitivity

D   Increase VP output

E   Increase ventricular blanking period

Answer

E Increase ventricular blanking period

Figure 63.3 Annotated tracing

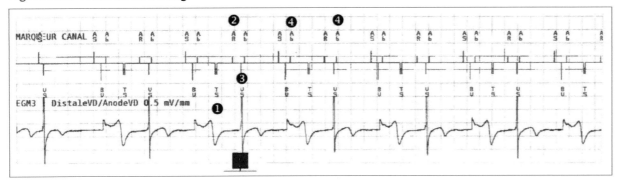

The patient has TWOS which leads to 2:1 biventricular pacing.

❶ TWOS falling in the VT zone (TS marker), at 370 ms from the biventricular paced (BV) event (Figure 63.3). The maximum programmable value for post-VP ventricular blanking in this device is 450 ms.

❷ The following sinus beat falls in the PVARP which is triggered by the preceding TWOS cycle, and is not tracked. Increasing atrial sensitivity would not solve the issue.

❸ Intrinsic ventricular conduction. Note that there is no TWOS with this cycle. Even if the PVARP had been shortened (and post-PVC PVARP extension inactivated), and the sinus cycle had fallen outside the PVARP, biventricular pacing would not have been delivered, due to limitation in the UTR (VS occurring at 390 ms from the tachycardia sense (TS) marker, corresponding to 60,000/390 = 154 bpm).

❹ FFRWs after biventricular pacing and VS, falling in the PVAB, without interfering with the timing cycles.

The TWOS algorithm (which was already activated) does not solve the issue, as it is only used for withholding inappropriate therapy upon detection of a VT or VF.

Comments

T-wave oversensing as a cause for reduction in CRT delivery

In this example (adapted, with permission, from Dayal et al.[1]), TWOS after biventricular pacing complex resulted in 2:1 non-tracking of sinus rhythm. It would not have caused inappropriate therapy, even if therapies had been activated in the VT zone, as *consecutive* tachycardia sensed events would be needed to detect VT, nor would this had been an issue if TWOS cycles had been detected in the VF zone, as the probabilistic X/Y counters would not have been satisfied.

The different options for troubleshooting TWOS in CRT devices are:

1 Increasing post-VP ventricular blanking, which does not compromise detection of ventricular arrhythmias as shorter refractory periods resume after sensed events (such as in the case of onset of VT/VF). The PVARP should also be extended as it should never be programmed shorter than the ventricular blanking period (see Volume 1, Case 24). In devices with adaptive ventricular sensitivity (such as CRT-Ds), ventricular blanking does not necessarily have to be programmed longer than the coupling interval of TWOS (Figure 63.4).

2 Adjusting dynamic sensitivity parameters. In some devices, the percentage of threshold start and/or delay to increasing sensitivity can be adjusted.

3 Reduce ventricular sensitivity. This may, however, compromise VT/VF detection.

4 Programming integrated bipolar sensing, which reduces TWOS. This is currently only possible in Medtronic devices. However, integrated bipolar sensing may increase the risk of diaphragmatic myopotential oversensing (see Volume 1, Case 45).

5 Programming LV-only pacing or sequential biventricular pacing. In the current example, TWOS only occurred during biventricular paced events. During fusion pacing resulting from the AdaptivCRT algorithm (see Case 67) no TWOS occurred due to the RV EGM being identical to that observed with intrinsic conduction (Figure 63.5).

6 Changing RV sensing lead. This requires intervening for repositioning the RV leads, adding a new pace-sense lead, or switching LV and RV leads for sensing.[2] The latter strategy is only possible if the patient has a bipolar (IS-1) LV lead and a DF-1 ICD lead. Furthermore, one cannot guarantee that TWOS will not recur with the new configuration.

Figure 63.4 TWOS occurs with the nominal ventricular blanking and adaptive sensitivity (bright red rectangle and line) and is avoided by increasing ventricular blanking (light red rectangle) to a value less than the TWOS interval, due to delay in onset of adaptive sensitivity (light red line), without changing the sensitivity level. Note that ICDs do not have a ventricular relative refractory period (only blanking); cf. Case 28

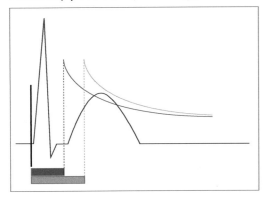

Figure 63.5 Absence of TWOS during LV-only fusion pacing (VP marker) by the AdaptivCRT algorithm in the present case. Note how the RV EGM is identical to that during the intrinsic conducted cycles (Figure 63.3)

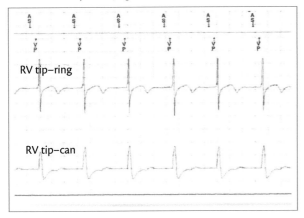

References

1. Dayal N, Burri H. T-wave oversensing: a cause of loss of cardiac resynchronization therapy. *Indian Pacing Electrophysiol J* 2016; **16**: 175–8.
2. Biffi M, de Zan G, Massaro G, Angeletti A, Martignani C, Boriani G, et al. Is ventricular sensing always right, when it is left? *Clin Cardiol* 2018; **41**: 1238–45.

Introduction to the case

During remote follow-up, a low percentage of CRT pacing was reported in a patient with a CRT-D device. Programmed parameters are shown in Table 64.1. The EGM of an episode of loss of biventricular pacing is shown in Figure 64.1.

Table 64.1 Device settings

Mode	DDDR
Basic rate	60 bpm
UTR	130 bpm
Maximum trigger rate	150 bpm
AV delay after pace	150 ms at 60 bpm and 120 ms at 130 bpm

Question

Figure 64.1 Transmitted EGM of an episode with interrupted biventricular pacing

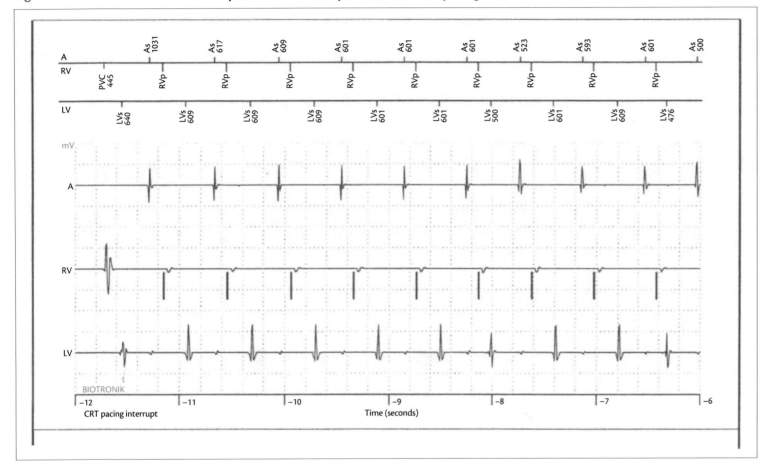

Which action can restore CRT pacing?

A Increase LV output

B Increase maximum trigger rate

C Increase RV output

D Increase ventricular blanking to 100 ms (maximum value)

E Shorten AVI

Answer

B Increase maximum trigger rate

Figure 64.2 Annotated EGM

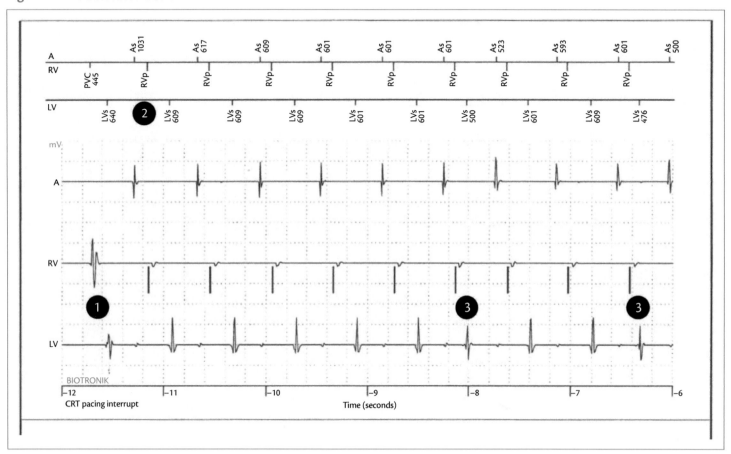

The EGM in Figure 64.2 displays left ventricular upper rate interval (LVURI) lock-in triggered by a PVC.

❶ Right-sided PVC sensed first in the RV channel and 195 ms later (640–445 ms) in the LV channel.

❷ RV pacing due to tracking of the AS event. This is possible as the PVC–RV pacing interval is longer than the URI for the RV channel. However, LV pacing is inhibited as this would violate the URI for the LV channel, given that LV sensing of the PVC occurred so late. This is then perpetuated for the following cycles due to the long interventricular conduction delay (approximately 220 ms) following RV pacing. Extending ventricular blanking to 100 ms would not solve the issue, but increasing the LV maximum trigger rate to 160 bpm would.

❸ These two beats are PVCs (probably left-sided as they are not visible on the RV channel). Note the change in EGM morphology and earlier coupling interval.

Comments

Left ventricular upper rate interval lock-in

This is a cause for non-delivery of biventricular pacing in Biotronik devices, which are capable of sensing via the LV channel (this is also possible with Boston Scientific devices, but is a rare issue due to a programmable ventricular refractory period of ≥250 ms, whereas ventricular blanking is only programmable up to 100 ms with current Biotronik devices). It is caused by the LVURI which inhibits LV pacing (Figure 64.3). The LVURI only inhibits LV pacing and does not impact right-sided DDD timing cycles.[1,2,3]

Figure 64.3 LVRI lock-in triggered by a PVC in the present case example, with depiction of right ventricular upper rate interval in blue (461 ms) and the LVURI in red (400 ms) corresponding to the programmed UTR of 130 bpm and maximum trigger rate of 150 bpm respectively. LV pacing cannot be delivered with RV pacing because of the ongoing LVURI, due to prolonged interventricular conduction times of the PVC and after RV pacing. Note that LV pacing is not triggered at the end of the LVURI

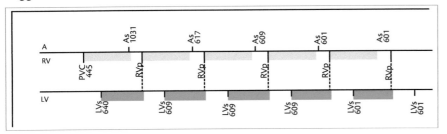

LV sensing was initially implemented to prevent LV pacing in the vulnerable period after a left-sided PVC with a very long interventricular conduction time and delayed sensing by the RV lead (i.e. before the depolarization wavefront reaches the RV lead and is sensed). However, proarrhythmia by LV pacing in this instance is highly unlikely as it will be delivered during the QRS of the PVC unless the delay is very long and sequential biventricular pacing with extreme RV pre-excitation is programmed, which is unusual, and will most probably result in non-capture of LV pacing and fusion with RV pacing. LV EGMs may identify lead integrity issues by revealing fracture artefacts, and also allow loss of LV capture to be identified (see Volume 1, Case 57). However, they add complexity to device troubleshooting by having to deal with unfamiliar timing cycles. In addition to causing LVURI lock-in, LV sensing may also withhold LV pacing due to far-field P-wave oversensing (if the LV sensing electrode is in a basal position of the coronary sinus tributary, see Volume 1, Case 66) or due to noise (e.g. pectoral myopotentials if sensing is programmed to unipolar).

LVURI lock-in is triggered by any situation which results in delayed LV sensing with a LVURI which is longer than the LV sensing–RV pacing interval. In addition to being triggered by right-sided PVCs with long interventricular conduction delays (or double-counting on the LV channel), it may be observed in case of loss of LV capture or in patients with LBBB with intrinsic AV conduction due either to atrial undersensing (Figure 64.4) or to heart rates which exceed the programmed UTR (Figure 64.5). In these instances, delayed LV sensing will result in retarded onset of the LVURI, with RV-only pacing, even once the heart rate falls below the UTR. Biventricular pacing only resumes once the heart rate interval exceeds the LVURI + interventricular conduction time.

Figure 64.4 LVURI lock-in triggered by atrial undersensing (*), resulting in the VS event being labelled as a PVC. Dashed lines correspond to RV events; solid lines correspond to LV events (LVp, left ventricular pacing; RVp, right ventricular pacing)

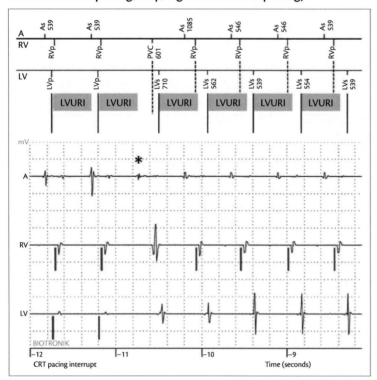

LVURI lock-in is maintained by long interventricular conduction delays after RV pacing, and fast heart rates. It can be avoided by increasing the UTR (which will avoid atrial non-tracking with intrinsic AV conduction) and also by decreasing the LVURI (by increasing the 'Maximum trigger rate' parameter). The 'Maximum trigger rate' parameter refers only to LV triggering and is by default set 20 bpm faster than the MTR (to a maximum of 160 bpm) to maintain LV pacing (Figure 64.5).

Figure 64.5 (a) LVURI lock-in resulting from intrinsic heart rate exceeding the UTR set to the same value as the maximum left ventricular trigger rate (MTR LV). Biventricular (BiV) pacing resumes only when the heart rate interval exceeds the interventricular conduction delay + LVURI. (b) When the MTR LV is set higher than the UTR, LV triggered pacing allows resumption of BiV pacing when the heart rate returns to the UTR

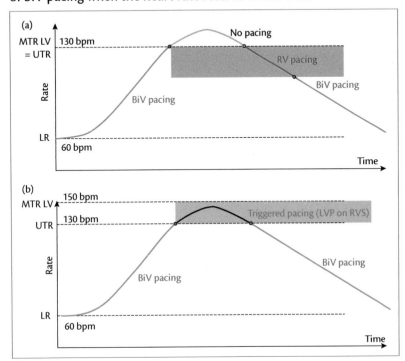

Another option is to inactivate the 'LV T-wave protection' function whereby the LVURI is only triggered by premature beats or LV pacing (and not LV sensing). Alternatively, LV sensing can simply be inactivated.

References

1. Barold SS, Kucher A. Understanding the timing cycles of a cardiac resynchronization device designed with left ventricular sensing. *Pacing Clin Electrophysiol* 2014; 37: 1324–37.
2. Haeberlin A, Ploux S, Noel A, et al. Left ventricular sensing in cardiac resynchronization devices-opportunities and pitfalls for device programming. *J Cardiovasc Electrophysiol* 2019; 30: 1352–61.
3. Haeberlin A, Ploux S, Noel A, et al. Causes of impaired biventricular pacing in cardiac resynchronization devices with left ventricular sensing. *Pacing Clin Electrophysiol* 2020; 43: 332–40.

Introduction to the case

A 45-year-old woman with non-ischaemic dilated cardiomyopathy, classified as NYHA class III, and reduced LVEF had been implanted with a CRT-D. During follow-up, an event classified as CRT pacing interruption was transmitted by remote monitoring and is shown in Figure 65.1. Device settings are shown in Table 65.1 and data on CRT pacing in Table 65.2.

Table 65.1 Device settings

Tachycardia		
Zone	**VT-1**	**VF**
Rate (bpm/ms)	181/330	207/290
Detection	32	30/40
Discrimination	On	
Therapy	Monitor	Shocks
Bradycardia		
Mode	DDD	
Base rate	60 bpm	
MTR	140 bpm	
Maximum LV trigger rate	160 bpm	
VP	LV – 50 ms	
AV delay	Paced	Sensed
At 60 bpm	140 ms	100 ms
At 130 bpm	90 ms	50 ms
PVARP	275 ms	
LV T-wave protection	On	

Table 65.2 Data on CRT pacing

CRT	
CRT pacing (%)	99
BiV pacing (%)	99
LV–RV sequences (only synchronizable events)	
BiV pacing (%)	99
RVp without LVp (%)	1
RVs triggered LVp (%)	0
RVs without LVp (%)	0
LVp exclusive (%)	0
LVp exclusive inhibited (%)	0
PVC triggered LVp (%)	0
PVC without LVp (%)	0

LVp, left ventricular pacing; LVs, left ventricular sensing; RVp, right ventricular pacing; RVs, right ventricular sensing.

Question

Figure 65.1 EGM of the transmitted CRT interruption episode

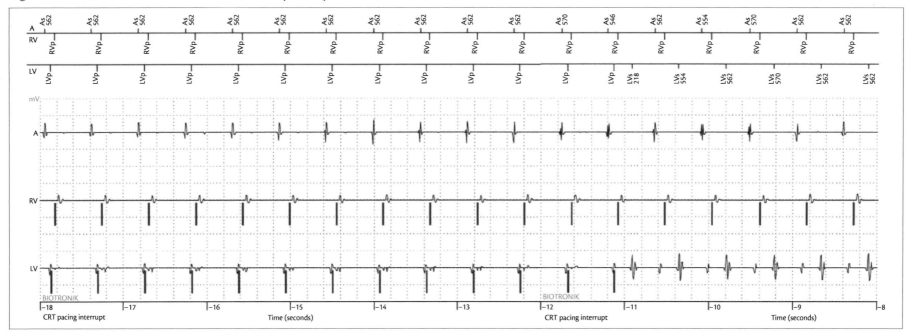

What is your diagnosis?

A Dislodgement LV lead

B FFRW oversensing

C Intermittent LV non-capture

D P-wave oversensing

E TWOS

Answer

C Intermittent LV non-capture

Figure 65.2 Annotated EGM

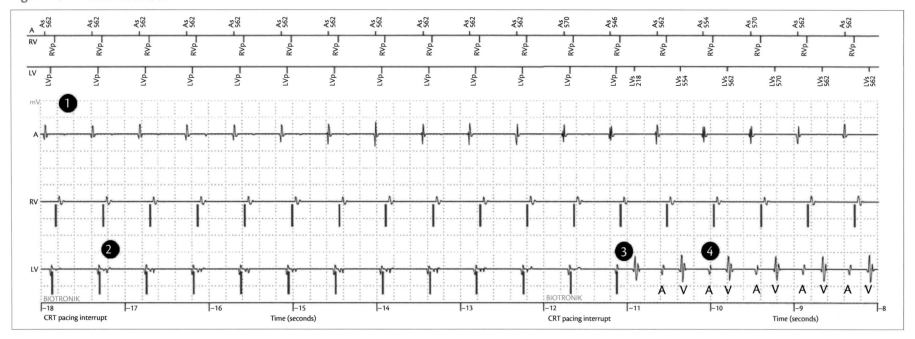

❶ Intrinsic atrial events with regular intervals of 562 ms (108 bpm), indicating sinus tachycardia (Figure 65.2).

❷ The LV EGM shows pacemaker spikes (blue vertical lines). Note, the two different EGM morphologies on the LV EGM. The small signal just preceding the pacing spike is caused by far-field P-wave (of the left atrium), which is, however, not sensed by the device (no corresponding markers). The 'fractionated' signal after the spike is caused by LV capture.

❸ LV non-capture; the high-amplitude signal on the LV EGM is LV activation caused by interventricular conduction after RV pacing. The two different morphologies described under ❷ are now clearly visible, atrial (A) and ventricular (V) activity separated by an iso-electric line.

❹ LV pacing is inhibited, as the interval from LVs 218 ms event to the next expected LV paced event (562 − 218 = 344 ms) is shorter than the programmed maximum LV trigger rate interval (60,000/160 = 375 ms, without accounting for small changes in the AVI related to differences in atrial cycle length between 546 ms and 562 ms). This then triggers LVURI lock-in.

Comments

Utility of left ventricular sensing to identify loss of left ventricular capture

This case illustrates how LV sensing can be useful for identify loss of LV capture, albeit with triggering of LVURI lock-in. Based upon the counters, this resulted in a 1% loss of biventricular pacing (RV pacing without LV pacing sequence). An option would be to inactivate LV T-wave protection, which would then not trigger a LVURI after LV sensing. However, loss of LV capture would then not be identified by LVURI lock-in with LV pacing interruption events.

Another option to identify loss of LV capture is for the device to evaluate LV EGM morphology (Figure 65.3).

Figure 65.3 Medtronic EffectivCRT diagnostic feature to identify loss of LV capture. Cycles with effective capture are identified by an initial negative deflection on the EGM (indicating spread of activation from the pacing site) and annotated by a 'Y' marker. Cycles with loss of capture are identified by an initial positive LV EGM (indicating activation propagating towards the electrode), and are annotated by a 'N' marker. Note the VVT mode indicated by the large oval with VS events triggering biventricular pacing (with pseudo-fusion), due to conducted atrial flutter. The algorithm analyses 100 consecutive ventricular events every hour and determines the percentage of effective LV capture

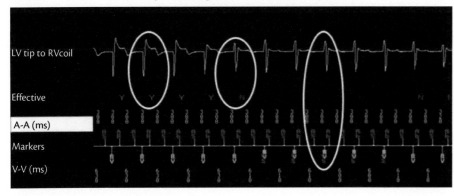

Reproduced with permission from Medtronic.

Introduction to the case

A 62-year-old man with ischaemic cardiopathy and LBBB had been implanted with a CRT-D for primary prevention of sudden cardiac death. An event classified as CRT pacing interruption was transmitted by remote monitoring. The EGM is shown in Figure 66.1. The device settings are shown in Table 66.1.

Table 66.1 Device settings

Tachycardia		
Zone	**VT-1**	**VF**
Rate (bpm/ms)	181/330	230/260
Detection	32	30/40
Discrimination	On	
Therapy	ATP + shocks	Shocks
Bradycardia		
Mode	DDDR	
Base rate	50 bpm	
MTR	150 bpm	
Maximum trigger rate	140 bpm	
VP	LV – 30 ms	
AV delay	Paced	Sensed
At 60 bpm	130 ms	90 ms
At 130 bpm	100 ms	60 ms
PVARP	225 ms	

Question

Figure 66.1 EGM of the transmitted episode

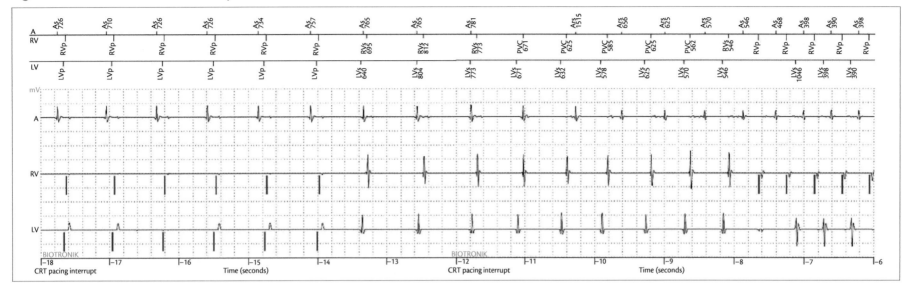

What is your diagnosis?

A   AT

B   Endless loop tachycardia

C   Non-capture of LV lead

D   Rate-drop response

E   Slow VT treated by ATP

Answer

B Endless loop tachycardia

Figure 66.2 Annotated EGM

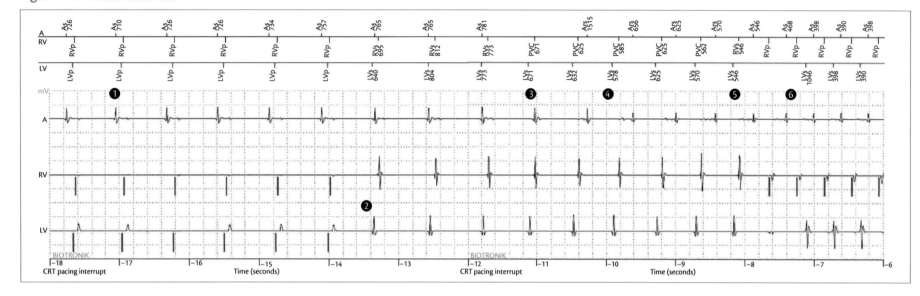

The tracing in Figure 66.2 shows a sequence of events leading to endless loop tachycardia with LVURI lock-in.

❶ Sinus rhythm, rate approximately 82 bpm, with tracked sequential biventricular pacing.

❷ Onset of ventricular rhythm which accelerates to slow VT (which is below the programmed VT-1 zone). Note that the EGM morphology and LV sensed–RV sensed sequence of this rhythm stay constant for the next eight cycles. The initial three cycles are not annotated as a PVC, as AS precedes RVS. Note that LVS does not affect right-sided timing cycles (the nearly simultaneous atrial event is sensed, as there is no PVAB, and the closely-coupled RV event is sensed, as LVS does not trigger a RV refractory period).

❸ Undersensed atrial activity due to cross-chamber blanking after RV sensing (PVC marker). The RV sensed event is now annotated as a PVC on the marker channel, as no atrial activity is detected preceding this event.

❹ Stable retrograde conduction can be observed (note acceleration of atrial activity to the ventricular rate). VA interval is approximately 200 ms. The retrograde atrial activation is detected in the PVARP (annotated as ARS on the marker channel).

❺ In Biotronik devices, RV sensed events preceded by AR sensed events which are within 350 ms are annotated as RVS (and as PVCs if the delay is >350 ms). A specific feature of these devices is that there is no PVARP after RVS (only after RVP or PVC events), and the following atrial sensed event is therefore labelled as AS. This starts an AVI, which is prolonged due to the MTR, followed by right ventricular pacing (RVP). There is no LVS signal or marker due to the analogue blanking period,[4] as RVP is synchronous with the hidden LV event. LV pacing is inhibited by the maximum trigger rate which is programmed at 140 bpm.

❻ Endless loop tachycardia (note AVI to the programmed value) with LVURI lock-in and RV-only pacing with an interventricular conduction delay of about 140 ms. This is not ATP as no VT episode was identified and atrial activity is being tracked. The PM-mediated tachycardia recognition algorithm would have terminated the tachycardia.

Comments

Knowledge of specific device features to fully elucidate a tracing

In this case example, the reader should have been able to recognize the endless loop tachycardia and correctly answer the question. However, to fully elucidate the tracing, detailed understanding of device behaviour is necessary. Specific features of all devices are difficult (if not impossible) to memorize but are usually available for reference in textbooks or in the manufacturer's technical manuals and online resources. In this example, the specific Biotronik features are as follows:

PVARP: only activated after VP or PVCs, and not after VS (contrary to other manufacturers).

Atrioventricular control (AVC) interval: this interval is used to identify device-defined PVCs. The AVC intervals starts with an AS event, an AP, and an atrial event sensed in the PVARP (ARS). The duration of the AVC interval is 350 ms and is programmable (250–800 ms) to avoid a PVC lock-in in patients with long PR intervals. A VS event in the AVC interval is classified as a non-PVC sensed RV event (RVS). A RVS event beyond the AVC interval is classified as a PVC.

LV sensing: currently only available in Biotronik and Boston Scientific devices. LV sensing was initially intended to avoid LV pacing in the vulnerable period after left-sided PVCs with long interventricular conduction delay and does not affect right-sided DDD timing cycles. However, this is theoretically almost impossible, because a left-sided PVC will result in a fusion beat with RV capture and non-capture by the LV lead (due to refractory myocardium). Pacing will always be delivered during the QRS complex and not on the T-wave, unless sequential RV–LV pacing is programmed (and even then, the LV myocardium is likely to be refractory due to the VV delay being limited to 100 ms).

LVURI: this is a separate upper rate interval for the LV and determines whether a LV pacing stimulus can be delivered.[1,2,3] LV pacing is cancelled if it falls in the LVURI. The duration of this interval can be changed by modifying the maximum trigger rate. An issue with this interval is the propensity to result in LVURI lock-in with RV-only pacing. Current devices have a maximum trigger rate programmed by default 20 bpm faster than the UTR. With the default UTR of 130 bpm (and maximum trigger rate of 150 bpm), LVURI lock-in will still occur if the interventricular conduction delay is >62 ms (corresponding to the difference in these rate intervals, i.e. 60,000/130–60,000/150), which is the case in most patients with LBBB or with RVP.

LV T-wave protection (LVTP): this feature determines in which circumstances an LVURI is started and is intended to prevent pacing in the vulnerable period of the T-wave. When LVTP is activated, an LVURI will be started by LV paced or sensed events. In case of deactivated LVTP, only LV paced events and right-sided PVCs will start an LVURI.

Zeroband feature (digital noise gating): this is a proprietary Biotronik feature designed to compress digital data and save memory space during recording of very low-amplitude signals (slightly lower than the programmed sensitivity of the channel), which will be automatically replaced by a zero line. Note the rectilinear aspect of the ventricular channels in Figure 66.2, which are explained by this feature (small signals are still visible in the atrial channel, due to the lower programmed sensitivity value).

References

1. Barold SS, Kucher A. Understanding the timing cycles of a cardiac resynchronization device designed with left ventricular sensing. *Pacing Clin Electrophysiol* 2014; 37: 1324–37.
2. Haeberlin A, Ploux S, Noel A, et al. Left ventricular sensing in cardiac resynchronization devices—opportunities and pitfalls for device programming. *J Cardiovasc Electrophysiol* 2019; 30: 1352–61.
3. Haeberlin A, Ploux S, Noel A, et al. Causes of impaired biventricular pacing in cardiac resynchronization devices with left ventricular sensing. *Pacing Clin Electrophysiol* 2020; 43: 332–40.

Introduction to the case

A patient with a CRT-D was seen at follow-up. The patient had no complaints. During the visit, the tracing shown in Figure 67.1. was observed. The EGM recorded in real-time during the event is shown in Figure 67.2.

Figure 67.1 ECGs recorded during in-office follow-up

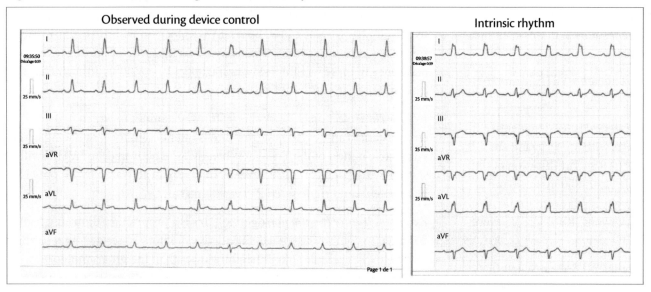

Question

Figure 67.2 Real-time EGM during in-office follow-up

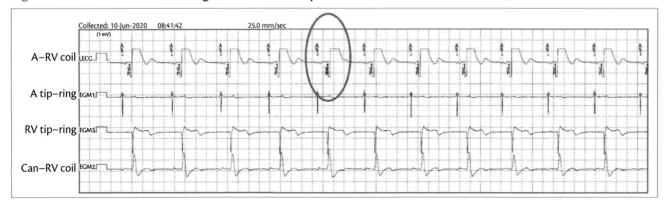

What do you observe (circled cycle)?

A Automatic ventricular capture threshold algorithm

B CRT optimization algorithm function

C R-wave double counting

D Ventricular premature beat

E Ventricular safety pacing

Answer

B CRT optimization algorithm function

Figure 67.3 Annotated tracing

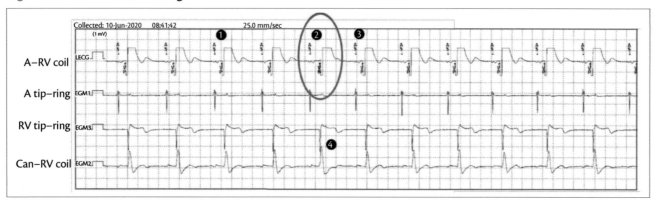

❶ The device is delivering LV pacing only (VP marker instead of biventricular marker) to deliver pacing which fuses with intrinsic conduction (Figure 67.3).

❷ The device measures the intrinsic AV delay every minute (with triggered VP to maintain some degree of CRT). Note the lengthened AVI.

❸ The programmed AVI is then adjusted based upon this measurement. In this instance, there is no noticeable change in the interval before and after measurement of the intrinsic AV delay.

❹ Note that the EGM on the near-field RV channel (RV tip–ring) is identical during cycles with LV pacing and during the conducted beat, due to local RV activation resulting from intrinsic conduction in both these instances. The far-field EGM (Can–RV coil) is, however, slightly different, reflecting changes in QRS morphology (Figure 67.1).

A shortened (and not lengthened) AV delay would be expected with an automatic capture threshold algorithm (to avoid pseudo-fusion), ventricular safety pacing (which only occurs after AP) or a ventricular premature beat.

Comments

Cardiac resynchronization therapy optimization algorithms

There is increasing evidence that fusion between intrinsic conduction and biventricular or LV pacing offers greater benefit than standard biventricular pacing.[1] There are a number of algorithms available that aim to synchronize VP and intrinsic conduction. One of these is the Medtronic AdaptivCRT algorithm, which is illustrated in this case, and the function of which is shown in Figure 67.4. Recent Biotronik and Abbott devices have an algorithm which functions in a similar manner, with programmable adjustments to the AV delay.

Figure 67.4 Function of the AdaptivCRT algorithm. The algorithm measures intrinsic AV conduction delays that are updated every minute during one beat (the VVT mode may maintain some degree of CRT) as well as P-wave and QRS durations measured on the far-field EGM (can to SVC coil or to RA ring), which are updated once every 16 h (during five consecutive beats, without VVT pacing). BiV, biventricular; LVCM, left ventricular capture management. * In models released as from 2016, the intrinsic AV delays that qualify for LV pacing are extended by 20 ms (i.e. from 200 to 220 ms for the sensed AV delay and from 250 to 270 ms for the paced AV delay)

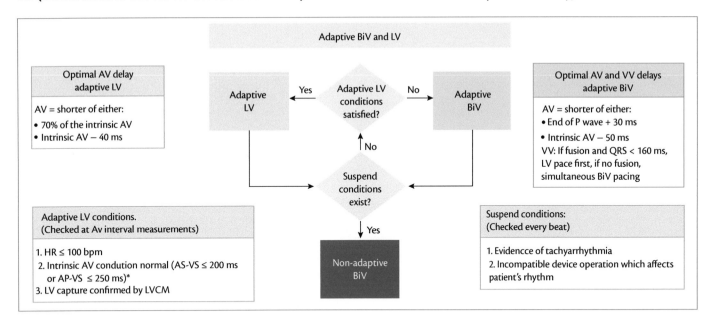

References

1. Burri H, Prinzen FW, Gasparini M, Leclercq C. Left univentricular pacing for cardiac resynchronization therapy. *Europace* 2017; **19**: 912–19.

Introduction to the case

A 62-year-old woman was admitted to the intensive care unit with acute pulmonary oedema requiring intubation. She had a past medical history of myocardial infarction with LVEF of 25%, NYHA class III heart failure, and LBBB for which an Abbott CRT-D had been implanted. The doctors on the intensive care unit were concerned as they saw intermittent loss of pacing spikes on telemetry. Her 12-lead ECG and device interrogation are shown in Figure 68.1.

Question

Figure 68.1 Screenshot of EGM during episode

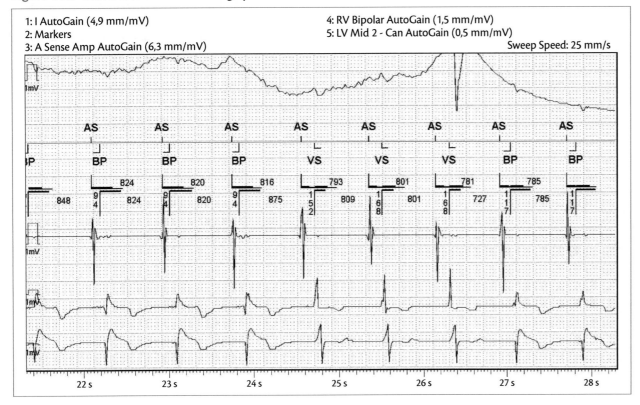

What explains the temporary loss of biventricular pacing?

A AV hysteresis algorithm to minimize VP

B AV optimization algorithm

C Intrinsic R-wave measurements

D Rate-adaptive AV delay

E Sensed AV delay programmed too long

Answer

B AV optimization algorithm

Figure 68.2 Annotated EGM

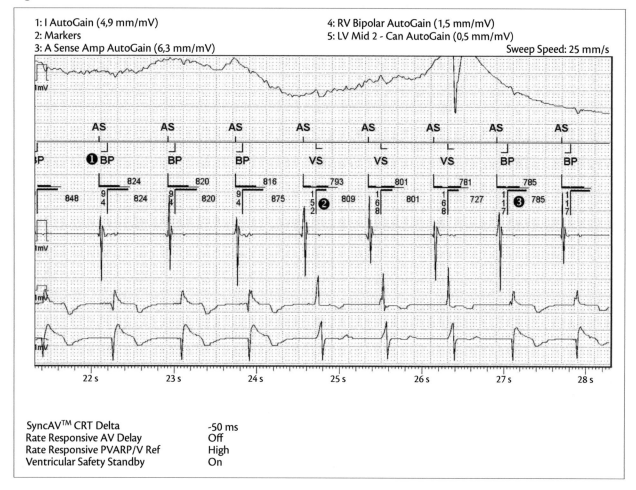

1: I AutoGain (4,9 mm/mV)
2: Markers
3: A Sense Amp AutoGain (6,3 mm/mV)
4: RV Bipolar AutoGain (1,5 mm/mV)
5: LV Mid 2 - Can AutoGain (0,5 mm/mV)

Sweep Speed: 25 mm/s

SyncAV™ CRT Delta	-50 ms
Rate Responsive AV Delay	Off
Rate Responsive PVARP/V Ref	High
Ventricular Safety Standby	On

❷ For three consecutive beats, biventricular pacing is omitted. This is part of an AV optimization algorithm, in this device named SyncAV. The algorithm omits biventricular pacing for three consecutive beats every 256 beats while the devices measures the AV delay. The programmed AV delay is then adjusted so that biventricular pacing is delivered with a predefined offset (SyncAV Delta). In this device the delta is programmed at 50 ms.

❸ The AV delay is reprogrammed to 117 ms (167 ms – 50 ms SyncAV delta). This allows fusion VP with activation from three distinct wavefronts: intrinsic AV activation, RV capture, and LV capture.

This cannot be part of a pacing avoidance algorithm as biventricular pacing would not have resumed following extension of the AV delay and successful intrinsic AV conduction. Furthermore, if it were automatic R-wave measurements, the AV delay would not have been adjusted. A rate-adaptive AV delay would shorten the AV delay as the heart rate increases. In this case, the atrial rate increases slightly yet the AV delay lengthens.

❶ Initial EGMs (Figure 68.2) demonstrate AS beats followed by biventricular pacing. There is successful capture on both the RV and LV electrodes as the EGM of both channels are simultaneous and different in morphology compared to the three cycles with intrinsic conduction. Note the 'QR' morphology in the unipolar LV EGM indicating local capture (and the 'RS' morphology with the three intrinsic cycles).

Comments

Cardiac resynchronization therapy optimization algorithms

In selected CRT recipients, well-timed negative AV hysteresis with fusion pacing with intrinsic AV conduction can reduce QRS duration compared to standard biventricular pacing.[1] Furthermore, in LBBB, RV activation may be normal, and LV-only pacing may be delivered to avoid inducing RV dyssynchrony. All devices which offer this feature have to periodically determine what the current PR interval is. This can be as frequently as every minute and can be measured over as little as one AV delay. In the current example, the Abbott SyncAV algorithm measures the AVI over three cycles to check for stability, and to avoid undue shortening of the adjusted AVI due to ventricular premature beats falling after an atrial event (see Volume 1, Case 63). The device will allow intrinsic AV activation to occur at the programmed long AVI and then shorten the AVI by the programmable offset. This allows tailoring of CRT programming to shorten QRS duration and increase CRT delivery in case the intrinsic AVI shortens over time (e.g. in case of reduction in beta-blocker dose).

Reference

1. Thibault B, Ritter P, Bode K, et al. Dynamic programming of atrioventricular delay improves electrical synchrony in a multi-center cardiac resynchronization therapy study. *Heart Rhythm* 2019; **16**: 1047–56.

Introduction to the case

A 60-year-old man presented to the pacing department for a routine device check 6 months following an implant of a primary prevention CRT-D. This was implanted for persisting severe LV systolic dysfunction due to aortic regurgitation, treated with a mechanical aortic valve replacement. He had NYHA class III dyspnoea and LBBB. His device trend graphs are shown in Figure 69.1 and a real-time EGM in Figure 69.2.

Figure 69.1 Device trend graphs

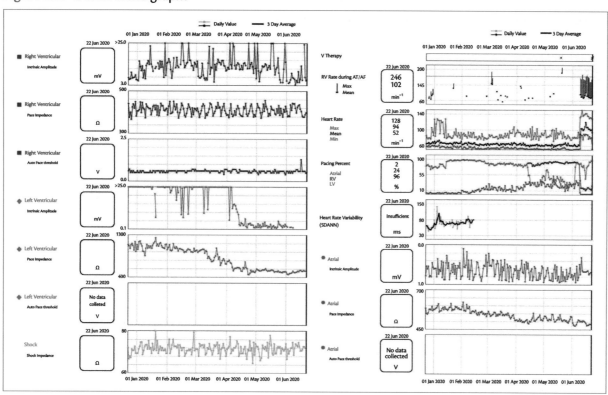

Question

Figure 69.2 Real-time EGM

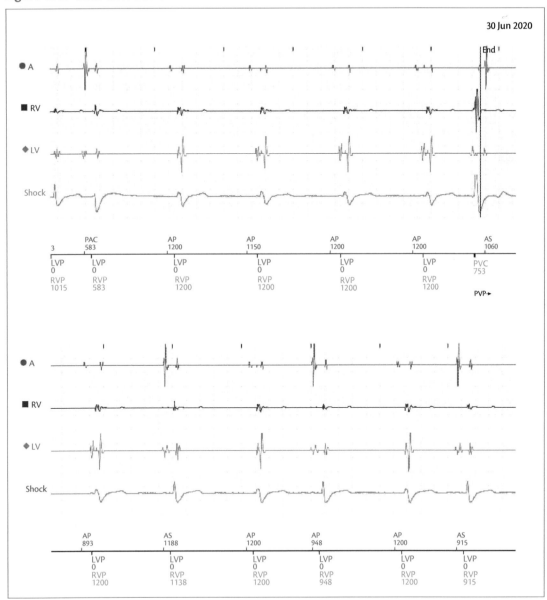

How might the problem be resolved?

A Increase pacing output of LV

B Increase pacing output of RA

C Reposition LV lead

D Reprogramme LV offset to pace LV first

E Shorten AV delay

CASE 69

283

Answer

C Reposition LV lead

Figure 69.3 Annotated EGM

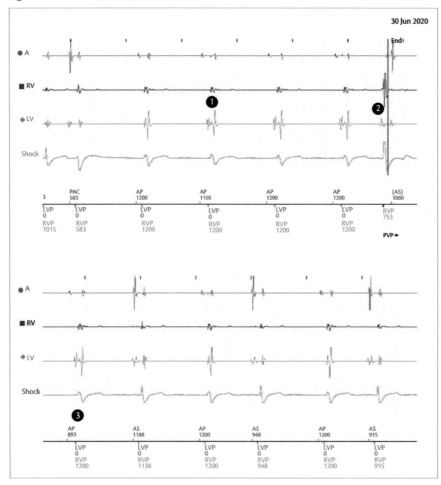

❶ The LV EGM (Figure 69.3) shows two signals. The first small signal shortly follows AS and AP events and corresponds to an atrial potential (which is not sensed). The second larger signal is synchronous with the LV pacing marker ('LVP') and corresponds to the ventricular signal.

❷ PVC visible almost simultaneously on LV and RV channels, and both early after the onset of the R-wave on the far-field channel, indicating that the LV lead is likely to be in close proximity to the RV lead and therefore not in the coronary sinus. Note the 'PVP→' marker indicating that the device has prolonged the PVARP following the PVC to reduce the likelihood of a PMT. The atrial signal is visible on both the atrial and LV EGMs.

❸ This device is operating on ventricular-based timing following VP events and PVCs. Note that AP is timed so as to deliver VP at the LRI of 1200 ms (50 bpm) —see Volume 1, Case 23.

Comments

Left ventricular lead displacement

In this case we can see that the LV EGM displays both atrial and ventricular signals. This occurs when the LV lead is implanted in a very basal position in the tributary vein (see Volume 1, Case 66), has displaced back into the coronary sinus, or sits across the tricuspid annulus. From the EGMs alone, we cannot be certain where the lead is positioned. There is, however, little/no lag between the ventricular signals seen on the RV EGM and LV EGM, it is therefore likely that the lead is straddling the tricuspid valve. Had it displaced into the coronary sinus, we would expect to see a ventricular potential after a delay resulting from RV capture and transseptal conduction. Furthermore, we would also expect the PVC to be sensed at different periods on the RV and LV EGM depending on which ventricle it originated from. Figure 69.4 shows lead position on the chest X-ray.

From the graph trends we see an acute drop in the LV R-wave measurements in mid-April which likely coincides with the lead displacement. We also see an acute drop in LV pacing percentage without a drop in RV pacing percentage. This is likely due to P-wave oversensing on the LV lead (which is not present in the current tracing). If the LV lead senses the P-wave, then subsequent ventricular depolarization will fall within the LV protection period. This is an interval (300–500 ms) following an LV sensed event, designed to avoid LV pacing in a vulnerable period if a left-sided PVC is not yet sensed on the RV lead (however, LV pacing in this instance will most probably not result in capture, as it will be delivered during the QRS of the PVC).

Figure 69.4 Chest X-rays showing lead positions at the time of implant (a) and at presentation 6 months later (b). The lead was subsequently replaced with an active fixation LV lead

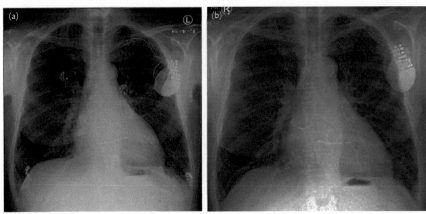

Introduction to the case

A patient implanted with a CRT-D underwent repositioning of a dislodged coronary sinus lead. On the day following the procedure, the VT event shown in Figure 70.1 was retrieved.

Question

Figure 70.1 Electrogram from the ventricular tachyarrhythmia event retrieved from the device memory

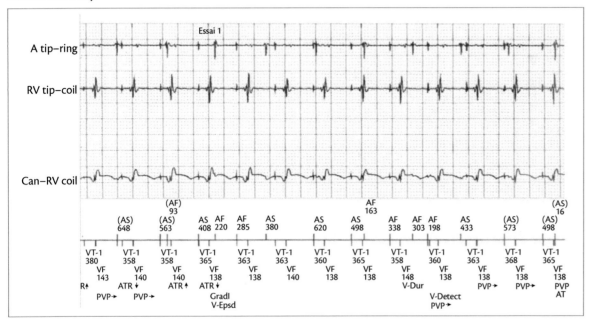

What is your diagnosis?

A Connector problem

B External EMI from an unknown source

C Far-field P-wave oversensing

D Lead chatter

E None of the above

Answer

E None of the above

Figure 70.2 Annotated tracing

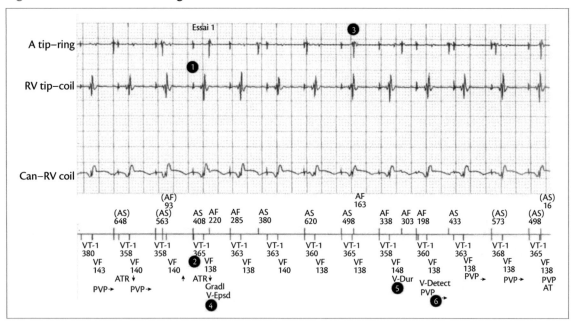

The event shown in Figure 70.2 results from the capture threshold test at implantation of the coronary sinus lead on the preceding day, using an external pacing system analyser. Antitachycardia therapies had been inactivated in the device, but not arrhythmia detection.

❶ The unipolar pacing spike delivered by the coronary sinus lead is visible in all three channels. Each spike is followed by a near-field signal on the RV channel detected after 138 or 140 ms, corresponding to the depolarization wavefront from LV capture reaching the RV lead EMI from an unknown source would not impact ventricular rhythm.

❷ A 'VT-1–VF' sequence is observed corresponding to sensing of the pacing spike and the near-field ventricular signal. The pacing spike is also detected in the atrial channel.

❸ Sinus rhythm is visible, dissociated from ventricular activity (i.e. the patient had VA block).

❹ A 'V-Epsd' marker is visible after 8/10 intervals falling in the ventricular tachyarrhythmia zone. This initiates the duration timer, during which ≥6/10 intervals of a sliding window need to fall in the tachycardia zone to keep incrementing the timer.

❺ After the programmed duration (2.5 s in the VF zone in this patient), a 'V-Dur' marker is seen.

❻ The episode is classified as a ventricular arrhythmia ('V-detect' marker) but no treatment is delivered due to therapy inactivation.

Comments

Unexpected findings after device implantation or revision

Devices can record events occurring during procedures and lead to puzzling findings. Another example is recording of ventricular arrhythmias during VT ablation, terminated by external ATP or defibrillation, or external cardioversion of AF, for which no event markers for treatment delivery will be displayed on the EGMs.

Index

Note: Tables, figures, and boxes are indicated by an italic *t*, *f*, and *b* following the page number.

291